EMBODY THE SKELETON
A Guide for Conscious Movement

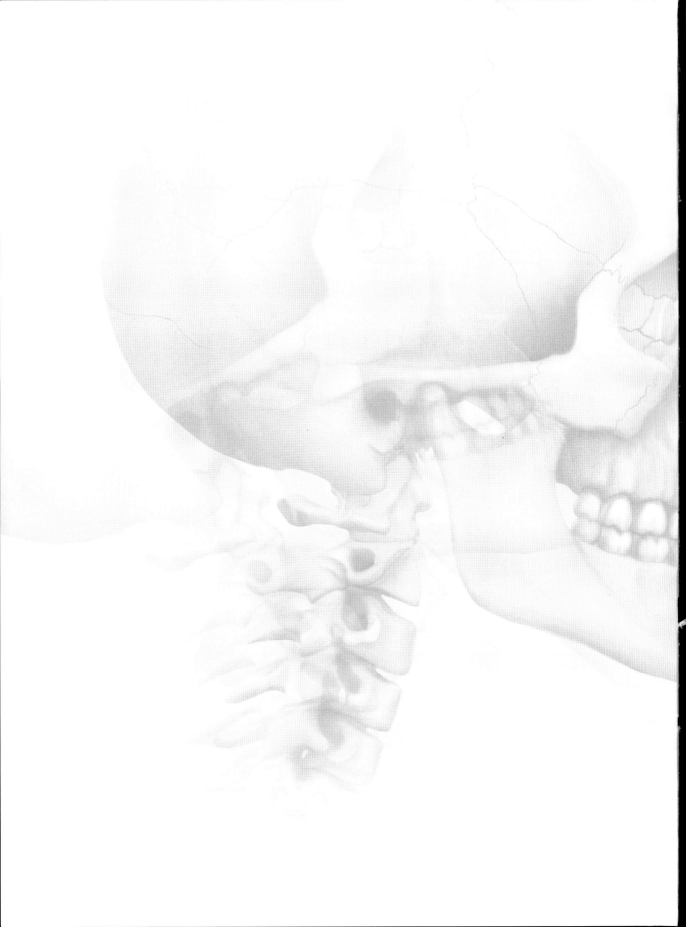

EMBODY THE SKELETON

A Guide for Conscious Movement

Mark C Taylor, RSMT
Director: Center for
BodyMindMovement
Pittsburgh, Pennsylvania, USA

Forewords
Martha Eddy, EdD
Don Hanlon Johnson, PhD

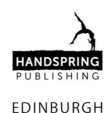

HANDSPRING PUBLISHING

EDINBURGH

HANDSPRING PUBLISHING LIMITED
The Old Manse, Fountainhall,
Pencaitland, East Lothian
EH34 5EY, Scotland
Tel: +44 1875 341 859
Website: www.handspringpublishing.com

First published 2019 in the United Kingdom by Handspring Publishing

ISBN 978-1-912085-09-5
ISBN (Kindle eBook) 978-1-912085-10-1

British Library Cataloguing in Publication Data
A catalogue record for this book is available from the British Library

Library of Congress Cataloguing in Publication Data
A catalog record for this book is available from the Library of Congress

Notice
Neither the Publisher nor the Authors assume any responsibility for any loss or injury and/or
damage to persons or property arising out of or relating to any use of the material contained in
this book. It is the responsibility of the treating practitioner, relying on independent expertise
and knowledge of the patient, to determine the best treatment and method of application for the
patient.

Commissioning Editor Sarena Wolfaard
Illustration and Design Emily Holden, Emily McDougall Art
Project Manager Jane Dingwall
Cover Art Shannon Carleen Knight
Back Cover Photography Enrique Meléndez Vargas
Indexer Aptara, India
Typesetter DiTech, India
Printer Melita, Malta

The
Publisher's
policy is to use
paper manufactured
from sustainable forests

Acknowledgments

My delight in movement awareness is rooted in my early training in dance and somatics. I am grateful to have been a student of Myra Avedon, Maggie Black, Judith Blackstone, Patricia Wittyk Boyer, Merce Cunningham, Kathy Grant, Melissa Hayden, Lucas Hoving, and Bessie Schönberg. Martha Myers, Dean Emeritus of the American Dance Festival, changed the course my life by guiding me toward somatic movement disciplines in a way that addressed both personal and professional needs. I am grateful to my first collaborators—most importantly Nancey Rosensweig, Donna Brandenburg Gangloff, and Mary Williford Shade—who taught me and explored with me, and to the many dancers who challenged and guided me as a choreographer: notably Gillian Beauchamp, Dennis Birkes, Lori Brungard, Barbara Canner, John Evans, Jennifer Keller, Peter Kope, André Koslowski, Michele de la Reza, Gwen Hunter Ritchie, Michael Walsh, and Andrew Wollowitz.

Embody the Skeleton originated in 2007 as a manual for the Center for BodyMindMovement. I thank Wendy Mackin and Jeri Lynn Anderson for their help, and Mary Lou Seereiter and Jan Cook for their valuable insights during its development. Elisabeth Osgood Campbell, Deborah Gouge, Ray Eliot Schwartz, and Lou Sturm helped immeasurably in transforming the book to its current form, and I am grateful as well for the support of Tim Vernon, Anna Thompson, and Taylor Knight. Steve Davies, Marie-Aimée de Montalembert, Leslie Apablaza Schmidt, and Ramiro Sanhueza generously provided me with space for thinking and writing.

Several individuals have been instrumental in the growth of BodyMindMovement in recent years, including Mariana Camarote, Sven Doehner, Julia Menéndez, Venerable Soorakkulame Pemaratana, and Stanley Perelman. I am inspired by and grateful for my current collaborators Debra Clydesdale, Rodrigo Palma, Diana Sánchez, Margery Segal, and Ivana Sejenovich, and the many students in BodyMindMovement training programs in Brazil, Ireland, Mexico, Oregon, and Pittsburgh. Elisa Cotroneo and the board of directors of the International Somatic Movement Education and Therapy Association work selflessly to grow the field of somatic movement. I am grateful to them, and those who nurtured the organization in the past, for holding an expansive vision for embodied movement and its impact on the world.

I thank my family, Barbara and William, for their love and support. Finally, my fascination with the body and mind in movement has been deeply influenced by Bonnie Bainbridge Cohen, the founder of Body-Mind Centering®. I once heard her say that "art in its finest moment is healing and healing in its finest moment is an art." That statement brought my world into focus and made sense of my life: I offer my profound thanks to her and the Body-Mind Centering® community for their vision and leadership in the field of somatic movement education.

Mark C Taylor, RSMT

Contents

Foreword

As teacher on the faculty of the School for Body-Mind Centering® (BMC) in the 1980s in Amherst, MA, I often considered revamping, for publication, the BMC Teacher Certification project that my long-time colleague Sara Vogeler and I developed. It is a pre-computer, hand-typed, detailed and revised manual on the skeletal system as viewed from the vantage of BMC. With the creation of this new 21st Century book—*Embody The Skeleton*—that particular project idea has definitely been postponed. The concept of embodying the skeletal tissue and its many purposes and functions has surely found its fruition in this book by Mark Taylor.

This book provides a much needed deeper analysis of, relationship with, and integration of, our physical "container," particularly our bones. Through clear writing, detailed drawings and practical activities you are taken on an elegant and intricate journey. Clear directives are provided on how to use movement, touch, visualization and awareness in experiencing one's bones and the articulations between them (the joints). Furthermore you are invited also to explore the movements and dances that are possible when truly embodying your skeletal structure.

The journey moves in a classic somatic direction from self-care to the care of others, guiding you to be gentle with oneself and also how to be caring and effective with students, whether in groups or in one-on-one sessions. I am personally grateful to be able to assign this book as a curricular support for the study of Dynamic Embodiment Somatic Movement Therapy—my 28-year-old blend of the work of Irmgard Bartenieff and Bonnie Bainbridge Cohen.[1]

In *Embody the Skeleton* Taylor has synthesized an approach to the teaching of skeletal anatomy that is totally in alignment (pun intended) with any of these three somatic movement trainings—Dynamic Embodiment, Laban/Bartenieff Studies and Body-Mind Centering®. In addition to this, it will be an asset to all other educational programs that seek to teach the anatomy of the skeletal system in an embodied way, using a somatic approach.

As you engage with this book know that you are getting much more than what is found in a traditional Anatomy & Kinesiology book vis a vis skeletal anatomy. You are being guided to feel the bones, move them with proprioceptive sensitivity, make sense of movement concepts that will support healthy functioning and to explore, if you choose, creativity and expression. Bones give us form and shape the nature of our interactions. How do they do this? Their specific make-up and dimensions define our body shape (or morphological type) and determine the directionality of movement, defining the ways that we can move. Everyone has variations in their personal skeletal structure—we therefore each are blessed, and limited, by these particularities. We also have personality. We each sequence muscles, bones and other body part usage in our own specific style. These components—morphology and personality—define how we can move. We can decide how we will move within these parameters. Decisions attending to the body and physical movement are most often unconscious. This book joins a lexicon of books that help you make more conscious your own movement habits and capacities. It will also help you find what directions are limited in your repertoire and/or your student's or client's. It has been said that form follows function. From this perspective, our human functioning, which in large part is determined by our personal movement choices, heavily influences our structure. What better way to improve skeletal health than to become astutely aware of both one's form and one's functioning. We can do this by more consciously choosing what we want to prioritize and make important. Embodiment helps in this process. It helps us become more conscious of our habitual choices, as well as our volitional behavior. *Embody the Skeleton* guides you through this process. Through awareness of your basic structure and your personal peculiarities (we all have them) you will come to understand more about how to access enhanced functioning—connecting your movement to meaning-making.

You may be asking how can bones move without our muscles? Well they cannot. Muscles pull bones and that is a fact. However, how we initiate movement can be nuanced in terms of what muscles contract when. My first somatic guides in the 1970s were students of Irmgard Bartenieff, physical therapist and developer of the first full certification curriculum in Laban Movement Analysis, training Certified Movement Analysts (CMAs). By 1978 I was studying with Bartenieff directly. Soon thereafter I had the privilege of assisting her on the certification faculty. Over these years she repeatedly stated that muscle action is complex, implying that it's unwieldy to attempt to be conscious of their sequencing of firing. She helped us to access our muscles in a different way. Bartenieff taught that muscles can easily be guided into clear action, by sensing the bones and establishing "spatial intention"through the bones (Bartenieff, 1980). The heart of Bartenieff Fundamentals involves learning bony landmarks—the protuberances we can easily feel on the surface of the body—in order to quickly picture and if desired, set intentions for our bones.

Once we know where our bones are to be directed in space the muscles needed to perform the action generally fall into place. The exceptions are when the muscles are greatly inhibited, unable to use their full range of contractility due to under or overuse. In this case, the bones once again can come to

the rescue—through imagery, clarity of joint action and practicing "skeletal initiation" muscle tensions can slowly subside and underused areas can gain strength. As you read through these chapters you will learn about the inner scaffold of the body, the skeleton and all its protuberances of import, and find multiple roadways to proper joint use which in turn help with relaxing muscles. The beauty is in the outcome—the experience of aligning bones in stillness and in action.

The story of the embodied skeleton has both roots and for sure a legacy. Bainbridge Cohen acknowledges Irmgard Bartenieff for having taught her the clarity of the bones,[2] as well as about the flow of movement and more (Bainbridge Cohen, 1993). Taylor cites Bonnie Bainbridge Cohen, founder of Body-Mind Centering® as a strong influence on his work, BodyMindMovement. These influences permeate this book and will make their way through his students and readers who are doing other somatic movement trainings. Each student will be assisted by the verbal and graphic visual aides as *Embody the Skeleton* becomes required reading for a plethora of somatic movement experts.

We can see its legacy in action in this one story of my own educational experience. Bartenieff first taught me the connection between the fingers and the different parts of the scapula (see page 138 in this book).[3] I was struck by learning this again when studying with Bonnie Bainbridge Cohen and how she had taken the work further by naming specific ridges of the scapula in relationship to fingers, and in making connections from the fingers to the ribs as well. Bainbridge Cohen went on to also name skeletal relationships between the toes and pelvis (as you will find described by Taylor on page 89).[3] Some years later I learned that Bainbridge Cohen had studied with Bartenieff. The development of ideas moves through generations. In *Embody the Skeleton* we are endowed with the lineage from Laban, to Bartenieff, to Bainbridge Cohen, to Taylor.[4]

And this is just one trajectory. Other great somatic movement educators also focused on the bones in intriguing ways, most particularly as pathways to improved health. Gerda Alexander, a contemporary of Bartenieff's in Germany, had her students embody the bones in order to balance the muscular tonus in the body. Fritz Smith of Zero Balancing, one of the most renowned osteopaths in the United States, developed protocols for healing bones and healing the body through movement of the bones.

The legacy of moving concepts and consciousness from teacher to students, through cultural milieus and paradigm shifts is the topic of my own book, *Mindful Movement: the evolution of the somatic arts and conscious action* (Eddy, 2016). Through the articulation of both new and evolving concepts, Taylor moves us forward as a community of seekers and educators. He begins with our structure, our skeleton, and how to embody it. He has cut a path for many more books to come.

Martha Hart Eddy, EdD
September 2018

Martha Hart Eddy, international speaker based in New York City, is the founder of Dynamic Embodiment Somatic Movement Therapy, which is affiliated with numerous universities around the United States. She is featured on network news for her somatic movement work with older adults and cancer patients called Moving For Life and author of *Mindful Movement: the evolution of somatic arts and conscious action.*

References

Bainbridge Cohen, B., 1993. Sensing Feeling and Action. Northampton, MA: Contact Editions.

Bartenieff, I., with Lewis, D., 1980. Body Movement: Coping with the Environment. London: Routledge Press.

Dowd, I., 1995. Taking Root to Fly. Northampton, MA: Contact Editions.

Eddy, M., 2016. Mindful Movement: the evolution of the somatic arts and conscious action. Bristol: Intellect Press.

[1] My earliest movement teachers were Tara Stepenberg, CMA, Diana Levy, DMT & CMA, Bonnie Bainbridge Cohen (1993), now a CMA, and Irene Dowd (1980, 1995) who taught at the Laban/Bartenieff Institute of Movement Studies. Each were privy to direct contact with Irmgard Bartenieff. Mark Taylor was indirectly influenced by his certification with Bonnie Bainbridge Cohen.

[2] Personal communication circa 1990.

[3] Taylor adds in the role of the forearm and foreleg in these connections.

[4] I'm delighted to report that I am part of this lineage having taught in the certification programs of Body-Mind Centering® from 1984–1994 and as a guest teacher ever since.

Foreword

While it is true that the map is not the territory, the overuse of this slogan obscures an equally important aspect of maps: their indispensible function in enriching our lives. I write this fresh from having experienced the great benefits of maps on a camping trip to the eastern Sierra Nevada where, following USGS contour maps, we found ourselves on an isolated campsite at 10,000 feet, above a river-laced meadow at the foot of a cirque of 13,000 foot peaks. From there, we spent a week exploring the countless glaciers, waterfalls, hidden canyons, carpets of wildflowers, inhabited by many living beings from elk, bear, eagles and osprey to butterflies and moths, and the myriad tiny insects. Having spent over half a century exploring the wilds of the world, I have accumulated many maps that have helped me navigate those once unknown places to find many of the riches lurking there that, without the maps, I might never have located.

Our bodies are like those awesome wilds of the natural world with its endless nooks and crannies, diverse materials of intricate shapes and densities, flows of different qualities and rhythms. But too often, well-meaning attempts to return to our embodiment lack the kind of maps that would lead us into the depths and intricacies. We are often given first-grade-like instructions to pay attention to our breathing, to feel our feet on the ground, to listen the sounds around us, without the specificity that would lead us into the actual territories of lungs, diaphragm, sinuses. While such simple kinds of directives do indeed make us aware that we are embodied beings, they are to the infinite riches of our bodies what a view of the Sierra Nevada from an airplane flying high above is to the revelations being gained by the hikers below.

Mark Taylor's book is like a high-quality USGS map geared for usage by serious explorers who are devoted to taking the time and care to take on the life work of finding out what is here. Beyond the elementary school strategies which survey the area from the generalized height, these practices carry the wanderer into strange shapes and interstices, whose unfamiliar contours yield new, and often healing, realizations about our lives.

But in addition to maps, an explorer of the high altitudes also needs to have some familiarity with the requirements of those unfamiliar regions: the sudden shifts of weather that can cause hypothermia or extreme dehydration. Because water sources are crucial, one needs to know something about purification. One needs to have the right clothing and sleeping gear, knowing of the enormous winds and sudden appearances of rain at that altitude. In the Sierra, one has to have bear canisters or the food supply will soon be dragged away in the night.

Mark's book fills a similar need in that it not only lays out the territory of our bones, but it also addresses the questions pertaining to the meaning of bones in our lives, the context in which it makes sense to devote oneself to exploring bones at such a depth. It also addresses the kinds of touch and sensitivities that an explorer has to cultivate if they are to succeed in navigating the many very different pathways through our bony selves.

This is such a valuable tool for this crucial task, a wonderfully skillful guidebook.

Don Hanlon Johnson, PhD
August 2018

Don Hanlon Johnson is the founder of the Somatic Psychology Program at the California Institute of Integral Studies in San Francisco and a professor in that program. His most recent book is *Diverse Bodies, Diverse Practices: Toward an Inclusive Somatics.*

Introduction

My moving, vital, physical body carries within it both the coded instructions for how to become human and the imprint of my particular experience of being alive. My life experience carries with it a unique set of joys and wounds that have shaped my body and mind, and determine how I move on the planet. When I focus with precise and fearless attention on my tissues and their movement I begin to recognize myself in depth, and my body is reminded of its native intelligence. This act of embodiment allows for transformation on physical, emotional, intellectual, and spiritual levels, facilitating change through the layers of my being.

As a practitioner of somatic movement education and therapy for 20 years and with 20 years' experience as a dancer, choreographer, and movement educator before that, I have personally used somatic movement to become a more accurate witness of my behavior and to become more fully myself in expression and relationship. As a somatic educator and therapist, I guide other people to be more expressive, more whole, and to move more easily in the world, both physically and mentally.

Based on my dance education experience and years of somatic movement studies with Bonnie Bainbridge Cohen and other somatic innovators, I started the Center for BodyMindMovement in 2007. This book originated as a manual for the first BodyMind-Movement skeletal course and has been enriched over the years by witnessing the experiences and hearing the insights of many groups of students. In these chapters, I invite you into the embodiment process through the lens of the bones. I offer it as a guide for your own embodiment and as a resource for sharing movement awareness with other people, whether friends, students, patients, or partners. If you are a movement teacher in dance, yoga, martial arts, or another movement discipline the information presented here can support you to refresh your conception of the body. For bodyworkers, manual therapists, or psychotherapists who want to include movement awareness in their repertoire it can serve as a handbook for new exploration. Based on the experience of those who have used the manual in the past, the process also resonates with people who are simply interested in personal growth. Whatever your application is for skeletal embodiment, I invite you first to come home to your own bones, and then to communicate to others the joy of living in theirs.

BodyMindMovement is one of a growing family of somatic movement disciplines that includes the Alexander Technique, Body-Mind Centering®, Continuum Movement®, the Feldenkrais Method®, Hanna Somatic Education®, and Shin Somatics®, among many others. These methods have developed through time, some arising spontaneously through the research of a founder and some passed orally and experientially through generations of teachers and practitioners traceable to the late 1700's (Eddy, 2016, p. 102). In addition to carrying the imprint of our direct lineages, many contemporary somatic movement disciplines draw on multiple traditions and integrate their work with related fields of interest, such as psychology, spirituality, traditional medicine, and the sciences (Eddy, 2016, p. 103).

The communication of somatic awareness from teacher to student is both an oral tradition and a creative process, which is what I hope to stimulate in each reader. The methodology of this book is based on that of Bonnie Bainbridge Cohen, which itself draws on many different lineages (Eddy, 2016, pp. 111-116). I have also absorbed and incorporated the wisdom of my earlier teachers in dance, the insights of my current teaching colleagues, Alexander and Feldenkrais principles, and studies in Buddhist philosophy, craniosacral therapy, developmental psychology, and Somatic Experiencing, to name a few. All of this experience has been filtered through my own imagination, so the work I share is and is not my creation: it is my individuated expression of an ongoing community inquiry.

Whatever the source, each somatic discipline provides multiple approaches for bringing internal subjective awareness to the experience of the body in movement. The process of cultivating conscious movement allows efficient movement patterns to replace inefficient ones and results in ease of movement, more responsive postural alignment, and the creation of space for internal reorganization where necessary. Bringing mindfulness to movement also allows the body's native intelligence to stimulate regenerative processes on cellular, tissue, and organic levels.

In BodyMindMovement, the cultivation of movement awareness assumes that the history of an individual's interaction with the natural, familial, cultural, and social environments impacts on habits of mind and movement. Those impacts, whether life-giving or traumatic, can resonate through and affect all tissues, organs, body systems, and developmental processes. We use awareness as medicine to reinforce the positive impacts and mitigate the negative ones, creating space where needed for the body to reorganize itself.

Each aspect of the self that we study—whether through structure, function, or imagination—is simply a lens through which we observe and enjoy a deepening connection with the body and the intelligence of its tissues. This book treats the skeletal system as that lens, but it is important to acknowledge that as we cultivate awareness in bone we are affecting all the neighboring tissues as well—the organ systems contained within bony cavities; the surrounding connective tissue matrix of fascia,

ligaments, and tendons; and the fluid, neuroendocrine, and muscular systems. We understand that the moving body is an integrated dynamic system composed of many interrelated parts. When we support conscious movement in one system of the body, we necessarily enrich and enliven all the others.

Enjoying the Skeletal System

Our individual living bones work together to provide our bodies with form and clarity in relationship to space. The joints between them provide articulation and movement. The resulting skeletal system provides both stability and mobility, creates a container for our organs and soft tissues, allows us to resist gravity while we move in space, and serves as the nursery for our young blood cells. Bones form the architecture of our body, and allow us to shape ourselves and reshape the world around us. Bone is alive and responsive, with the capacity to change shape in response to the pull of gravity, the tension of muscles, and the influence of sensitive touch.

By sensing its bones, the body can refine its relationship to gravity and establish an easy flow of weight through the joints. When the skeleton is allowed to do its work, the soft skeleton of the fascia and other supporting tissues are able to release unnecessary holding. Muscles no longer need to provide support but can perform their roles as mobilizers of bone. With a sensate skeleton, the entire body is free to move in response to the invitation of the environment.

In my experience, one feature of skeletal embodiment is that it organized me in space, providing awareness of such basic features as head to tail connection, core to extremity relationships, and bilateral symmetry. Embodying these skeletal relationships provided me with an enhanced sense of organization at the deepest levels of my being. As an example, we look at how the skeleton seeks the support of the earth before it moves in space. Without grounding through the bones, one's movement would be somewhat limited. This principle is mirrored in early life, when the nurturing support of parents and family provides a necessary precedent for psychological movement and growth. Children who lack that early support require compensatory effort to develop. What is true for the bones—that support precedes movement—is mirrored in the child's development.

Some years ago a client came to me saying that she felt lost, anxious about her place in the world. Throughout her adult life, her image of personal security had been that of someday having a house with a white picket fence. After some weeks exploring the skeletal system, she told me that by finding the sensation of her bones she had found her home. When she embodied her ribs in particular, she found that they provided her with the protection she craved. She knew that she had found safety, a home with a white picket fence within herself: she no longer needed to find a house in the suburbs to give her a sense of security. This book is intended to be a guide for you to come home to your bones, to find safety in them as she did.

Tools for the Embodiment Process

The tools for the journey of skeletal embodiment range from naming and categorizing the bones and their parts to basic kinesiology to experiential explorations of touch and movement. As you move through the skeletal system, you should expect to enjoy and embody the following ideas, knowledge, and principles. Ideally, you will be able to communicate them verbally, as well as through touch and movement, to other people.

Skeletal Anatomy

You will:

- Be able to identify all the bones in your body
- Understand bone as part of the connective tissue matrix
- Participate in the cycle of life within your bone
- Distinguish among the different types of bone.

Skeletal Kinesiology

You will:

- Be able to analyze movement in the spatial planes
- Be familiar with joint classification
- Be familiar with skeletal terminology.

The Bones in Movement

You will:

- Be able to initiate movement from the shafts of the bone and from the joints
- Differentiate among the three layers of bone and initiate movement from each of them
- Be able to initiate movement from the axial and appendicular skeletons
- Utilize the design of the skeletal system for both stability and mobility
- Enhance the equanimity of your joint spaces
- Embody lines of connection from the toes to the pelvis and from the fingers to the scapula
- Differentiate distal from proximal movement
- Originate distal movement at a joint from proximal support and proximal movement from distal support.

Touching the Bones

You will be familiar with the following hands-on practices:

- Mapping the bones with light touch
- Releasing bone from myofascial binding
- Awakening the three layers of bone
- Compression and release of joint spaces

- Sequencing compression through the bones
- Supporting equanimity within the joint space
- Facilitating passive range of motion in the joints.

Vibration in Bone

You will:

- Experience cellular respiration in your bones
- Sound into your bones.

Taking Skeletal Embodiment into the World

You will:

- Be able to organize a hands-on session with skeletal themes
- Be able to utilize skeletal principles in pedagogy.

Safe Touch in Partnering

Touching hands are not like pharmaceuticals or scalpels. They are like flashlights in a darkened room. The medicine they administer is self-awareness. And for many of our painful conditions, this is the aid that is most urgently needed.

– Juhan, 2003

All touch requires movement, from the subtle molecular vibration of cellular touch to the gross motion of releasing bone from myofascial binding. As we work with conscious touch in the skeletal system, we create space through which those who are touched can move more fluently, and those who touch can be reminded of their own vitality and inner movement.

Touch is one of the most powerful tools we have for initiating awareness and transformational process in the bodymind. When we touch specific tissues with clear intention, we have the capacity to awaken and release the flow of joy and connectedness. We also have the capacity, however, to awaken the residue of painful experience and trauma. When touch is not used with delicacy and compassion, it can be experienced as intrusive or dangerous.

When you are in relationship through touch, several basic principles will provide safety for you and your partner. These principles are equally important in educational and professional settings.

The Relationship

Remember that each relationship through touch is a duet. One person is more active and the other is more receptive, but you are both active participants responsible for yourselves and each other.

Humility

When you touch, you are not a healer; you are simply providing the awareness and space for your partner's body to reorganize itself. You are providing the guidance that brings awareness. Given the infinite complexity of the human body, there is no way that we can know what the other person needs. You are in a relationship, and through your embodiment skills you can provide a framework for mutual exploration. Always share your perceptions as observations that require mutual assessment, not as fact.

Innocence

Try to enter each session with an unbiased mind and a sense of not knowing. Try not to impose your ideas on the other person. Your work is an inquiry, and what you learn should be learned together. Each time you work with someone, start innocently and do not presume that you are doing something to them. Your deepest wisdom has the potential to emerge from a commitment to curiosity, to not knowing.

Compassion

Many people have feelings about, or problems with, touch, and it is helpful to know what your partner's comfort zone is before you begin. Be curious and sensitive to your partner's attitudes about touch based on their personal, cultural, and social background. Establish the ground rules for touch before you begin.

Comfort

Make sure that you are physically, mentally, and emotionally comfortable as you work. If you are holding tension, distress, or discomfort, this will be communicated to your partner. It is always best to take the time to shift your body for comfort, to articulate your feelings, or to describe your confusion, and let the awkwardness be an opportunity for deeper meeting.

Guidelines for Safe Touch

Work with the following list as a set of guidelines for touch:

- Know that you are touching the whole person when you touch any part of the person.

- Contact your own breath before starting and mentally honor yourself and your partner.

- Establish a clear moment of contact, knowing when the partnership in touch begins.

- Begin with non-judgmental touch.

- As in a dance, know when you are following your partner and when you are leading.

- Permit your partner and yourself to stop touch at any time.

- Stay in communication: you both should feel free to give feedback and to ask questions at all times.

- Encourage your partner to request changes in the style or type of touch.

- If you are the person giving touch, you are the more active participant in this duet. Take responsibility for maintaining communication.

- At the end of the session, provide a clear ending to touch, a clear separation, and mutual closure.

Safe Communication

In somatic movement education, verbal communication and appropriate feedback are just as important as safe touch in creating a relationship between partners. As a somatic guide, you are responsible for maintaining communication during a session and providing feedback in a helpful way. In professional settings, students or clients may not initially be aware of the importance of their feedback to you, so it is helpful to discuss both the guidelines for safe touch and the following guidelines for feedback with new students, clients, and partners.

Providing Feedback

Feedback is most helpful when it is spoken as an "I" statement. When receiving touch, it is more helpful to say, "I need a lighter touch" as opposed to the accusatory "Your touch is too heavy." As the one giving touch, it is more helpful for you to observe, "I feel some resistance in this area," rather than to say, "You are tight here." An "I" statement opens dialogue. The definitive judgment leaves no room for response, and creates a condition that may or may not exist. Try not to say anything that would limit possibilities for your partner, or assume that your perception through your hands is a reality for that person.

Receiving Feedback

When providing touch, listen to feedback nonjudgmentally. Your partners' needs do not necessarily have to do with what you are doing in the moment, and their feedback reflects their histories, prior experiences, and personalities. Their statements, even if clumsy, are useful information. Welcome them as guideposts for adjusting your attention to the specific dance at hand. Each communication from your partner has something to offer you, whether it is a confirmation of how you are working or an opportunity to try something different. Notice how and where in your bodymind you resonate with your partner's statement.

Ask for feedback and stay in communication!

Skeletal Embodiment in Context

It is very clearly apparent from the admonitions of Galen how great is the usefulness of a knowledge of the bones, since the bones are the foundation of the rest of the parts of the body and all the members rest upon them and are supported, as proceeding from a primary base. Thus if any one is ignorant of the structure of the bones it follows necessarily that he will be ignorant of very many other things along with them.

– Massa, 1559

All the bone in your body is alive and breathing! We are culturally conditioned to equate bone with death, through the omnipresent skeletons of Halloween and countless uses of skeletal imagery around the world, from Mexico to India. Many people become averse to the idea of working with bone simply because of its association with decay and dying. That is unfortunate because they lose out on experiencing the sensitivity of living, breathing, fluid bone. Living bone is completely unlike the dry remains after death. It is composed of living cells, nerves, fat, collagen, lymph, and fluids. In fact, according to Mitchell in the *Journal of Biological Chemistry* (Mitchell, 1945), your bones are 31 percent water. They are not stiff, but malleable, and readily change their shape based on the way you use your body.

Think for a moment about the history of your bones. Where have they been broken or bruised? What habitual activities do you perform that contribute to the shaping and reshaping of your bone structure? Which joints are happy and which are not thriving? Where is your bone structure thick and strong, and where is it more delicate and vulnerable? Because of its responsiveness, your skeleton is

unique to you, bearing the imprint of your life, your habits, and your style of being in the world. With all these things in mind, what is the personality of your skeleton? How does it express who you are?

Why Begin with Bone?

The embodiment of bone enhances the functional organization of movement in the entire body. Experientially I have found that the skeletal system is a great place to start a relationship with conscious movement, because it seems easier to re-pattern the movement of my body through bone than through any other single system.

For many years in my training as a dancer, I simply used my body as a tool, trying to shape it externally into a form that was demanded by traditions of dance technique and the requirements of the movement I was asked to perform. As a late-starting dancer, that approach made it difficult to improve technically. Relating to my body as an object to be tamed actually seemed to limit my progress. When I began to add somatic movement disciplines to my training regimen—especially those that worked from a skeletal perspective—I was quickly able to increase my technical proficiency.

Bone is the densest and most concentrated tissue of the connective tissue and musculoskeletal systems, providing the framework for everything else. When I experienced the sensation of balanced weight flow and relationships among my bones, my fascia was willing to adjust, my ligaments tended to balance and realign themselves around my joints, and my overworked muscles automatically retrained themselves to support more efficient movement pathways with less tension and greater reciprocity.

Why is that so? It may take science a long time to answer that question, but my experience is that paying attention to the proprioceptive and kinesthetic awareness of bones and their joint spaces stimulates plasticity in my brain and nervous system. As I focus awareness on my bones and joint spaces, my body becomes more willing to change than when I attempt to initiate change from my muscles or when I simply repeat movements in the hope that they will improve. Muscles are brilliant at repeating their actions, but less apt to change their habits of movement from within themselves. Like members of a football team, muscles need information from a coach to coordinate a response to a new stimulus, the opposing team. The team, working together as a whole, can then succeed, whereas individual players making many small changes might lead to disaster. My bone–brain relationship is an effective coach for the muscles.

Re-patterning the moving body occurs when we are able to listen deeply to the sensory stimuli of gravity, space, and changes of position in the bones and joints. Inviting these sensations to arise through bone seems to create a cascading effect in the nervous system that allows it to adopt new movement strategies quickly and efficiently. The argument is not that bone is the only way or the even best way for everyone to re-pattern movement, but that it is an efficient and pleasant way to begin the journey of conscious, mindful movement.

Now it is time to begin the process. This book contains numerous suggestions for explorations of the skeletal system through movement, touch, and observation. Some can be done alone and others require partners. The explorations are like scores for you to improvise upon: take what you like and use your imagination to expand upon them. The book is meant to stimulate curiosity, not to be the final word: take advantage of the wonderful resources in anatomy texts, other books, and the internet to widen and deepen your embodied understanding. Another suggestion is to read and record the explorations and let the playback be your guide rather than trying to remember the sequence or process. Several of the guided meditations in this book have been recorded as examples for your work. They are noted in the text with QR codes: scan the code on an internet-connected device and it will link to an online recording on the website *www.bodymindmovement.com* that you are free to stream or download.

Movement Exploration: Living in Your Bones

Make yourself comfortable, standing, sitting, or lying down, and change position whenever you like. Prepare by following your breath for some time and letting the weight of your body begin to settle toward the earth.

Bring awareness to the bones of your head, both facial and cranial. Imagine them softening, so that they feel much more fluid than normal, and even malleable. Focus your breath into the facial and cranial bones, and allow movement to arise from the sensation of relaxing, breathing, and feeling their fluids. Are you able to feel the relaxation of the soft living tissue of your jaw? Of your cheekbones? Of the bones around your eyes? Of the bones of your cranium?

Invite those sensations to flow down your vertebral column; take time to enliven the bones of your neck, thorax, lumbar spine, and sacrum. Imagine all the living bones of your spine a little juicy, a little resilient, and filled with breath and fluids. Notice the reactions in your body. How do your organs react? Your muscles? Your nerves?

Bring your attention to the bones of your hands and feet. Let them give your extremities form, but think of them as breathy and spongy. Imagine that water is able to travel through them, and notice how they choose to move when you focus on them in that way.

Invite that same quality into the bones of your forearms and lower legs. Then allow your upper arms and thighs to soften and enjoy the vitality of their living bones. Bring the sensation into the bones of your shoulders and pelvis, and notice whether your body gravitates toward movement or toward stillness as you introduce the sensation of living bone into your entire body.

Contents and Container

Any work of art needs to balance its form—the container—with its content, which is the heart of the matter and what is being communicated. Composers study musical form and a variety of structural elements (such as melody, harmony, and rhythm) in order to express their joy, anger, and other drives inventively. Choreographers employ the containing formal and structural elements of space, time, and energy to allow their bodies to express the content of the work: the idea, emotion, or impulse that is asking to be expressed.

My body itself is a work of art designed by deep evolutionary processes and my ancestral and personal interactions with the environment. It has elements—my container—that give me form. It also has elements within—my contents—that sustain my life and allow me to feel and express desire, love,

hunger, and satisfaction. My contents give meaning to my form, and my container enables my contents to express themselves.

Which parts of my body are central to my being? Which parts of my body enable that which is me to act in the world? The skeletal system and most of the rest of our connective tissue (ligaments, tendons, fascia, cartilage, and fat) form protective wrapping, padding, and receptacles for other tissues, in addition to providing architectural form for the body in space. That is the container system. Our organs, glands, and immune, fluid, and nervous systems are contained within these structures. They are the systems that comprise our contents.

Our container and contents systems are not separate; each depends upon the other for existence, like the principle of yin and yang. They are complementary, interconnected, and mutually dependent. Although the focus of this book is the skeletal system, you will be invited to notice the effects of the work with bones upon your entire being. The central nervous system, the organs, and the glands have a spatial, locational relationship with the axial skeleton, situated in the trunk of the body. As you refine your awareness of the curves of your spine, movement will begin to free your brain and spinal cord, and you will have access to sensory information flowing from the cord and its surrounding fluids. Not only will skeletal movement improve, but also there will be more space for your nervous system to function. Additionally, adjustments to the alignment and movement of your spine will create space for easy movement and function of your pelvic, abdominal, and thoracic organs.

In qigong we work with evenly distributing weight through the skeleton, giving me a strong feeling of being grounded. We also work with the idea that the bones are neutral whereas the fascia and skin hold the residue of tension, etc. from emotions. When I need to prevent myself from reacting to emotional triggers, I visualize the neutral quality of the bones.

— Greenleaf, 2017

Conversely, you may find that increasing awareness of your contents will support your skeletal function. For instance, I might observe the power of the fluids within my bones, feeling the expanding and condensing movement of cellular fluid as I breathe into my skeleton, the movement of blood through my bone, or the delicious mobilizing influence of synovial fluid between my joints.

I might use the embodiment of my central nervous system to provide integration to my spine, or the awakening of my peripheral nerves to lighten and revitalize the bones of my extremities. I can use the tone of my digestive tube to provide stability for the anterior surface of my spine, or the gliding of serous fluid between my organs to enhance spinal mobility.

Movement Exploration: Contents and Container

Touch your skull with your fingers to enliven the sensation of the bones. Initiate movement of your head in space from that sensation and begin to move the bones into your hands. Then allow the bony skull to explore space around you in every direction: this is moving from the container.

Then imagine that the space inside your skull is like a gigantic empty cathedral. Allow your breath to be the wind moving within the space. Let it flow front and back, side to side, and up and down. Allow the movement of the wind inside to move your head in space, and notice how different it feels to do that than initiating movement from the bones.

Gradually allow the cavity of your skull to be filled with the weight of its fluids, fats, connective tissue, and brain cells. Let the movement of your head now be initiated by the weight of your brain and its fluids. The movement may even take you to the floor: there you can roll your head, initiating from the organ weight inside. Allow the movement to take its time and to originate from the sensation of your fluid and weighty brain: this is moving from the contents. Compare the sensation of moving from the contents to how it felt to move from the container.

Shift your attention so that your ribs, sternum, and spine are the container, moving first from the bones and their many articulations, then moving from breath circulating within your chest cavity, and finally moving from its contents, the heart and lungs.

Finally bring awareness to the bony cavity of your pelvis. Touch the bones then initiate movement from the sensation of the container and its joints. Circulate breath within the pelvic and abdominal cavities, feeling the huge internal space, and enjoy movement that originates from breath. Finally move from the contents of your pelvis and abdomen: find pleasure in sliding, condensing, and expanding the digestive, reproductive, and urinary organs within.

Touch Exploration: Contents and Container

With your partner in a side-lying position, touch the ribs, spine, and sternum. Maintaining an awareness of the container, gently move your partner's body and feel the quality of movement that arises from the bony container.

Then invite your touch to deepen and become aware of your partner's heart and lungs. Drop your intention through their bones and initiate movement within the chest cavity, gently moving your partner's heart and lungs to initiate changes in position and movement in space.

Ask your partner to reflect on the quality of touch and movement initiated from the container compared to touch and movement initiated from the contents.

Observation: Contents and Container

Observe other people in stillness, and notice the variation in expression. Which ones express a sense of their container system? Which project a sense of their contents? In which individuals does there seem to be a balanced relationship between contents and container?

Observe people in motion and become aware of the variation in expression. Which ones initiate movement from their container system and project a sense of their form? Which move more from the contents and project a sense of their depth? In which individuals does there seem to be a balanced relationship between contents and container? For example, I have noticed that many children walk and run supported from an expansive vitality in their organs. Contrast that with the movement of an aging adult whose internal spaces seem saggy or lack vitality. The adult's contents may seem constrained as effort is embedded in musculoskeletal holding of the shoulders, pelvis, or other structures of the container.

Movement Constellations and the Bones

Movement is life, and life requires movement. As long as we are living, we are in motion, whether at a minute cellular level or enjoying movement in space—running, walking, sitting, breathing, dancing, cooking, or playing an instrument. In BodyMind-Movement, our study of bones is integrated with the study of the history of life on earth as expressed through movement, and the ways in which that history manifests in us as individuals.

A movement constellation is an aggregation of primitive reflexes, righting reactions, and behavioral responses that is the underpinning of the developing nervous system (Bainbridge Cohen, 2018). We highlight and work sequentially with a series of movement constellations that together are the basis for the full dimensionality of volitional human movement. As humans, our moving bodies reflect and contain all the stages of motor development as they occurred in deep time. Yet they also reflect the particularity of ourselves as individual manifestations of life.

Movement constellations include both fluid-based, oceanic patterns and the ones that emerged later with the development of a bony spine, first in the ocean and then on land. The ocean constellations provide fluidity, the potential of renewal, and a sense of connection to ones inner being. The land-based movement constellations provide greater specificity in movement and the increased ability to connect with and act on the environment. As animal life left the ocean, the density of bone became even more crucial in supporting the gravity-defying movement sequences necessary for the evolution of life on land. The movement constellations progress sequentially from one to the next, with the earlier and simpler ones supporting the more complex anti-gravity constellations that follow. We carry within ourselves the history of life, and our bones reflect the complexity of that history.

Two major shifts in our beings arose when we moved from the ocean onto land. The first is that all of our land-based movement occurs in relationship to gravity and space, giving us the experiences of weightedness and lightness. Unless you have the privilege of traveling in outer space, every moment of your life is spent in a dialogue with the pull of the earth. How you enter into that dialogue is fundamental to your movement, your health, and your enjoyment of life. The other shift arising from the need to deal with gravity is the increased complexity of body organization, which allows you to push yourself away from the earth and organize yourself functionally and creatively in a terrestrial environment.

All of your voluntary actions are based on specific constellations of movement through the bones of your body—spinal sequencing, symmetrical limb sequencing, same-sided limb sequencing, and cross-body sequencing. Embodying your bones helps to refine the series of constellated movements, providing greater strength, buoyancy, agility, and ease in your body as it relates to space and the earth.

The Basics (of Bone)

Before exploring specific bones within the skeletal system, it is important to develop a common vocabulary about the movement and formation of bone. Here we introduce the basic function, structure, and terminology of bone.

The Functions of Bone

It is important to remember that bones play many roles in our bodies. The most important functions include the following:

Support

This could also be called the structural function. Bones create a framework for the rest of the body by providing the architecture of the body in relationship to space and points of attachment for muscles.

Protection

The bones create safe spaces for our organ systems, such as the brain within the skull and the heart within the bony thorax.

Movement

Using joints, muscles lever the long bones, creating locomotion in space.

Mineral Homeostasis

Bone tissue stores and releases calcium, phosphorus, and other minerals as needed to support mineral balance within the body.

Blood Cell Production

The red marrow within our bones produces red blood cells, white blood cells, and platelets.

Energy Storage

The yellow marrow within our bones is an important reserve of energy in the form of adipose (fat) cells, which can be transformed into energy to be used by the whole body.

Endocrine Function

Bone secretes the signaling molecule osteocalcin, which modulates glucose homeostasis and contributes to the production of testosterone.

Bone Tissue

Our bones are composed of connective tissue, one of the four types of tissue in the body. (The others are muscle tissue, nerve tissue, and epithelial tissue or skin.) Connective tissue is the most abundant tissue in the body. It binds together, supports, and gives form to other body tissues, protects and insulates internal organs, and compartmentalizes structures such as skeletal muscles. Qualities of connective tissue include density, strength, elasticity, boundaries, resilience, wrappings, fluid connectivity, protection, padding, and adhesion.

All connective tissue, including bone, is composed of a matrix of living cells widely separated from each other. The matrix, which is created and sustained by the cells, is composed of fibers such as elastin or collagen and a ground substance. The ground substance can be fluid, semifluid, gelatinous, fibrous, or calcified, as is bone. The predominant fiber in bone is collagen, which is tough and resistant to tensile forces, yet allows flexibility. If you dissolve the minerals from a chicken bone in vinegar for a couple of days, what remains is the flexible, fibrous part of the matrix. You can then bend the bone easily.

Living bone consists of a complex system of living cells, each one with a different function in the life cycle of bone. In an adult, the skeleton replaces itself every ten years, meaning that ten percent of your bone mass is regenerated every year. Four types of bone cells contribute to this cycle of birth and death:

- Osteoprogenitor cells are precursor cells to other bone cells, and are found in the periosteum (the skin of the bone) and the endosteum (an inner lining). They are able to undergo mitosis or reproduction.

- Osteoblasts form bone by secreting collagen and other components of bone tissue, but they cannot reproduce.

- Osteocytes, mature cells that have developed from osteoblasts, are the principle cells of bone tissue. While osteoblasts form the bone tissue, the osteocytes perform the ongoing metabolic functions of sustaining the bone.

- Osteoclasts complete the cycle of bone growth and death, by absorbing and recycling the matrix, enabling the bone tissue to grow, reform, and repair where necessary.

Joint Classification

There are three functional classifications of joints, based on the degree of movement available:

- A synarthrosis is a minimally movable joint. Examples are the roots of the teeth within the sockets of the jaw; the sutures between the bones of the skull; and the joint between the first rib and the sternum.

- An amphiarthrosis is a slightly movable joint, such as the pubic symphysis and the articulation at the ankle between the tibia and fibula.

- A diarthrosis is a joint that moves freely. Its bones are covered with articular cartilage that cushions the bones and allows them greater resiliency; it possesses a joint capsule, which protects the joint and helps to direct and restrain movement; and it has a synovial cavity, or a fluid-filled space.

There are several sub-categories of diarthroses:

- Gliding joint, in which the articulating surfaces are flat, and movement is limited. Examples are the joints between the carpal bones.

- Hinge joint, in which the convex surface of one bone articulates with the concave surface of its neighboring bone. An example is the knee.

- Pivot joint, in which a rounded projection of one bone fits within a ring formed by another bone, permitting rotation around the axis of the rounded projection. An example is the atlanto-axial joint.

- Ellipsoidal joint, in which the oval condyle of one bone fits into an elliptical cavity of another bone, permitting movement in two planes. An example is the wrist joint.

- Ball and socket joint, in which a rounded head fits into a concave cavity, permitting free movement in all directions. The shoulder and hip joints are examples.

- Saddle joint, in which the opposing surfaces are reciprocally concave and convex, allowing all movements except axial rotation. The best example is the carpometacarpal joint at the base of the thumb formed by the trapezium and the first metacarpal.

Anatomical Terms and Orientations

A specialized vocabulary serves to clarify the location of and relationships among bones within the body. It is helpful to use these terms consistently when we study the skeletal system so as to be clear. These words describe directions, not places, so they are used with a specific or implied relationship to another body part.

The Language of Location, Direction, and Relationships in the Body

Distal	Farther away from the center of the body or midline
Proximal	Closer to the center of the body or midline
Core	The center or the trunk, as a point or region
Anterior	Toward the front surface of the body
Ventral	Toward the front surface of the body
Posterior	Toward the back surface of the body
Dorsal	Toward the back surface of the body
Medial	Toward the center or midline of the body
Lateral	Away from midline of the body
Superior	Closer to the head
Inferior	Closer to the feet
Cranial	Within the trunk, closer to the head
Cephalic	Within the trunk, closer to the head
Caudal	Within the trunk, closer to the tail
Superficial	Toward the surface of the body
Deep	Lying underneath

Bone Terminology

Specialized terminology allows us to name features that are common to many bones and joints.

Projections that are Sites of Tendon and Ligament Attachment

Crest	A narrow ridge of bone
Line or linea	A ridge that is less prominent than a crest

Spine	A sharp slender projection
Process	A protruding aspect of the bone
Ramus	A process extending like a branch from a larger bone
Trochanter	An unusually large and irregular process on the femur
Tubercle	A small rounded projection
Tuberosity	A large rounded projection or roughened area
Epicondyle	A raised area or prominence above a condyle

Processes that Help to Form Joints

Condyle	A rounded articular prominence
Head	A rounded extension of a bone carried on a narrower neck
Facet	A smooth, flat surface

Depressions and Openings Within Bone

Fissure	A narrow slit-like opening
Foramen	An opening through a bone, often round or oval
Fossa	A shallow depression in a bone, which can be part of a joint
Meatus	A canal-like passageway
Sinus	A depression or cavity within bone

The Body in Space

In order to observe, describe, and analyze the movement of the body in space and the functions of specific joints, it is important to have a vocabulary that accurately reports those motions. The following definitions, derived from the spatial analysis of Rudolf Laban (Bradley, 2009), are fundamental to understanding how our bodies move.

Directions

A direction is a line that starts at any point in space, proceeds to another point in space, and continues indefinitely. When working with the body, we identify six major directions, with the initiating point located at or near the center. The directions are up and down, left and right, and front and back.

Dimensions

A dimension is a combination of two directions with a common initiating point traveling opposite to each other. When working with the body, the major directions combine to form the dimensions. The up and down directions together form the vertical dimension. The left and right directions together form the horizontal dimension. The front and back directions together form the sagittal dimension.

The dimensions are consistent from the perspective of our bodies, no matter what our position is in space. The vertical dimension is defined by the central axis of the body, the spine, and is aligned with the spine whether we are standing, lying down, or leaning at an angle. Up is always a continuation of the direction of the head and down is always a continuation of the direction of the tail, no matter where our head and tail may be.

Planes

A plane is a combination of two dimensions. A plane can be thought of as something like a sheet of paper, if the paper did not have discreet edges and continued forever. The third dimension is missing from a plane and forms the axis for movement at a joint.

When we are analyzing movement of the body, the dimensions combine to form three planes: sagittal, vertical, and horizontal. These planes (Figure 2.1) are named after the dimensions, but are not to be confused with the dimensions. They are fundamentally different.

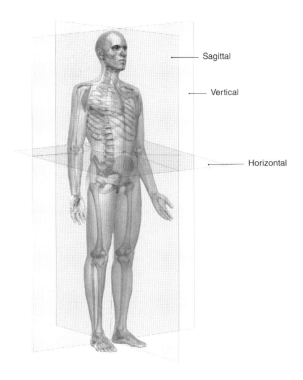

Figure 2.1

The planes

The Sagittal Plane

The sagittal dimension and the vertical dimension together form the sagittal plane. This is also called the wheel plane, because if you were standing behind a rolling wheel, the plane described by the wheel would bisect your body into right and left sides. The missing dimension, the horizontal, forms the axis for the sagittal plane.

The Vertical Plane

The vertical dimension and the horizontal dimension together form the vertical plane. This is also called the door plane, because if you were standing in a doorway, the plane described by the doorframe would bisect your body into front and back. It is also

called the coronal plane. The missing dimension, the sagittal, forms the axis for the vertical plane.

The Horizontal Plane

The horizontal dimension and the sagittal dimension together form the horizontal plane. This is also called the table plane, because if you were standing near a table, the plane of the tabletop would bisect your body into upper and lower parts. The missing dimension, the vertical, forms the axis for the horizontal plane.

Just as the dimensions of the body remain related to the vertical axis when we shift our position in space, the planes, which are defined by those dimensions, remain related to the body's vertical axis. For example, if you are lying on the ground, the vertical plane of your body is lying down with you. The matrix of space within the body remains consistent no matter what our position is relative to the earth.

Movement in the Planes

The description of movement in the planes is determined relative to a neutral starting position, called anatomical position. You can find anatomical position most easily by standing or lying supine (on your back). In either case, your spine is elongated, your toes and legs are directed forward, and your palms are open to the front. The descriptions below are all from anatomical position.

Movement through the sagittal plane (Figure 2.2) is called flexion when the angle of the joint is reduced when seen from the front of the body. Movement through the sagittal plane is called extension when the angle of the joint is increased when seen from the front of the body.

Movement of the spine in the vertical plane (Figure 2.3) is called side bending or lateral flexion. Movement of the limbs in the vertical plane is called abduction (movement away from the midline of the body) or adduction (movement toward the midline of the body).

Movement in the horizontal plane (Figure 2.4) is called rotation. We always rotate in reference to the longitudinal axis of the spine or the limbs. With regard to the spine, we distinguish between rotation to the right and rotation to the left. With regard to the limbs, we speak of internal (medial) or external (lateral) rotation.

Qualities of the Planes

Each of us lives in the three-dimensional matrix of space, and moves through the world differently from everyone else. Our personal movement habits develop through the way we relate to the earth and space with weight and lightness; through patterns of relationship with family and other people; and through our history of relationship with the environment. We habitually emphasize some planes more than others. Each plane carries with it a

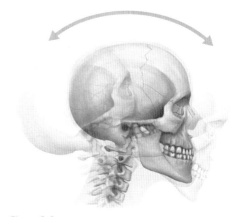

Figure 2.2

Movement in the sagittal plane

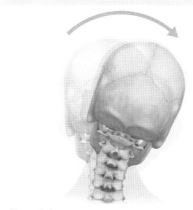

Figure 2.3

Movement in the vertical plane

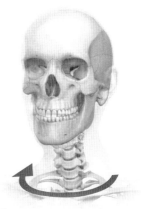

Figure 2.4

Movement in the horizontal plane

distinctive "mind," or quality of attention and perception. Watching the way we move in the planes can reveal much about our history and preferences. The ability to identify and perceive the way a person moves in the planes is an important diagnostic tool in somatic work.

The Sagittal Plane

The sagittal plane runs through the center of the body, front to back, and separates and balances the left and right sides. The flexion and extension patterns of sagittal plane movement produce a sense of doing, of action—specifically advancing or retreating. Advancing can have many qualities from attacking to approaching. Retreating can be defensive or deferential. Flexion of the spine is protective: a coming into self. Extension of the spine is expansive: a yield into space. We use upper-limb flexion to bring food to the mouth and thereby nurture ourselves. We use upper-limb extension to throw darts, projecting ourselves and objects into space.

Characteristics of movement in the sagittal plane include action, locomotion, protection, aggression, and withdrawal.

The Vertical Plane

The vertical plane runs through the center of the body, side to side, separating and balancing the front and back. It brings the front of the body into balance with the back of the body. Empsizing the side bending patterns of vertical plane movement provides an experience of taking in and processing information, rather than doing something or relating to others. Our ears are on the sides of the body; listening is a vertical plane activity! I can widen or narrow my legs from the hip joints, making an angel in the snow, but I can't walk without including sagittal plane movement. I can raise and lower my hands and arms to the side, up to the sky, but I can't bend my elbows or rotate my wrist to bring me into relationship with something. Those limitations actually give me space for noticing what is going on around me.

Characteristics of vertical plane movements include listening, assessment, attention, discrimination, analysis, taking in, planning, and presentation.

The Horizontal Plane

The horizontal plane separates upper from lower, balancing movement above and below a joint. The rotation of movement away from midline in the horizontal plane allows us to direct our intention into relationship with the environment and with others. Think of an infant turning her head to find the nipple, or a man looking over his shoulder to see who's coming from behind. As movement around the central axis develops it differentiates the lower body from the upper body and in a limb, it differentiates distal from proximal. Functionally, this differentiation in the horizontal plane supports curiosity and the ability to move into relationship. Horizontal plane movement allows me to twist a doorknob, to adjust my grip for a handshake, or to change the direction of my walk, my gaze, and my attention.

Characteristics of horizontal plane movements include communication, coming into relationship, giving and receiving, and engagement.

Movement Exploration: The Planes

Stand with your palms and toes facing forward, your feet directly under your hip joints. This is anatomical position, the reference point for analyzing movement.

Sagittal Plane Movement

Allow your spine to move in flexion and extension, enjoying movement in your cervical, thoracic, and lumbar regions, but not allowing side bending or rotation. Add your arms and legs, bending them and straightening them, but not allowing for rotation or widening and narrowing. If you are very strict, you will add your eyes, not letting them roam to the sides! See what you can do when you allow yourself only to flex and extend—be careful not to rotate your palms. You will probably be able to move forward and back, but not adjust your path, should you come toward someone or something. Notice what the feeling is of moving in the sagittal plane. How inventive can you be given the limitation? Notice how your mind works, and what would be easy and what would be difficult to do using this movement. This is the plane of moving into action.

Vertical Plane Movement

From anatomical position, invite your spine to flex laterally to each side, and limit any flexion/extension or rotation that may want to creep in. Begin to add widening and narrowing of your arms, fingers, legs, and toes, noticing which joints will help you widen and narrow and which won't. Hint: knees and elbows cannot move in the vertical plane! Notice the limitations of the movement, but find what your body can do when it is restricted to the vertical plane of movement. Notice how your mind works as well. This is the plane of assessment and discrimination.

Horizontal Plane Movement

From anatomical position, allow each segment of your spine to rotate to the right and left, enjoying movement in your cervical, thoracic, and lumbar regions, but not allowing flexion/extension or side bending. Add rotation in your arms and legs, enjoying the sensation of moving toward and away from midline. Notice what happens to your sense of self as you move with rotation, and how you begin to relate to the environment. If you are with other people, notice whether you are now able to make rotary adjustments to communicate with them a little more easily. Enjoy entering into and leaving relationship with them. This is the plane of communication.

Moving through the Planes

Before you finish, take some time to enjoy moving dynamically in all the planes. How many different actions can you get your body to do at the same time? How do you feel moving through all the planes? What happens to your breath, and to the tone of your muscles? Notice what feels strange to you and what feels familiar. Do your movement habits favor one or more of the planes?

Skeletal Embodiment: Movement, Touch, and Vibration

The tools presented in this chapter invite you explore the delicious mobility of skeletal system as a whole without limiting awareness to specific bones. Some use touch, others are movement based, and a few utilize sound and vibration. Explorations and principles that are specific to particular joints and bones are addressed in later chapters.

Embodying Axial and Appendicular Skeletons

The axial skeleton is the grouping of bones that forms the central axis of the body. The appendicular skeleton forms the limbs. In traditional anatomy, the axial skeleton includes all the bones of the head and skull; the vertebrae, sacrum, and coccyx; the ribs; and the pelvic bones. The traditional view of the appendicular skeleton is that it includes the shoulder girdle and arms, the hyoid bone, and the bones of the legs.

From the perspective of embodied movement, it is much more helpful to define the axial and appendicular portions of the skeleton based on function. The questions we want to address with this redefinition include:

- What is the functional unit of the central axis?

- What are the appendages that allow us to ambulate, reach, grasp, and feed ourselves?

- How do the axial and appendicular skeletons (Figure 3.1) relate to other body systems, particularly the nervous system?

From this point of view, we observe that the pelvic half participates in movement of the leg as a unit, starting at the sacroiliac joint. The ribs move with the arms in reaching out and gathering in. Similarly, the facial bones of the head help us engage in the tasks of taking hold of and releasing food, much as the arm does with objects, as well as gathering visual and other sensory information from the environment.

Therefore, from a functional perspective, the axial skeleton includes only the sacrum, the vertebrae, and the cranial bones, conforming to the idea that the axial skeleton is the protective space for the central nervous system—the brain and spinal cord. Functionally, the appendicular skeleton is formed by the facial bones and the jaw; the arms, shoulder girdle, and ribs; the pelvic halves and the legs; and the coccyx, which is a mobile appendage of the sacrum. From this perspective, the appendicular skeleton aligns more closely with the map of the peripheral nervous system, the nerve pathways that are situated outside the brain and spinal cord.

The axial skeleton, associated with the central nervous system, relates to inner awareness, perceptual processing, and the sense of self. The appendicular skeleton, associated with the peripheral nervous system, relates to the external world, with all the pleasure and pain elicited by moving into and feeling the environment.

QR Code #1: Axial and Appendicular Skeleton

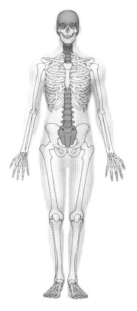
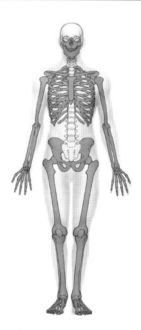

Axial skeleton   Appendicular skeleton

Figure 3.1

Axial and appendicular skeleton

Rolling Exploration: Axial and Appendicular

Roll across the floor of a room or studio, initiating movement only from the axial skeleton, using flexion and extension, rotation, and side bending of the vertebrae, cranial bones, and sacrum. Allow your extremities to dangle from the spine. Notice how and when the extremities might want to initiate, based on your personal habits. How does limiting the movement to your axial skeleton make you feel? What qualities of movement emerge?

Roll across the floor again, this time initiating movement from fingers, toes, tail, and eyes, and eventually from knees, elbows, and mouth. Allow multiple patterns of movement to emerge as you combine various body parts to initiate the movement. How does rolling in that way make you feel? In what way does it change your relationship to space and to yourself?

Standing Exploration: Axial and Appendicular

In standing, initiate movement from your spine and cranial bones. Invite weight and fluidity as you include awareness of the brain and spinal cord within the bones. Alternate spinal movement with movement initiated from your appendicular skeleton. Trace the peripheral nerve pathways up and down your arms and legs, leading away from and toward your spine, as you move your extremities. Which way of moving feels most familiar to you: axial or appendicular?

Work with patterns of condensing and expanding movement, traveling through space and different levels. As you do, allow the axial skeleton to support your appendicular skeleton and the appendicular skeleton to counter support your axial skeleton. Can movement flow equally through both?

Axial and Appendicular Movement with a Partner

In standing, explore the possibility of moving with a partner while both of you move only your axial skeletons. What are the possibilities, and what do you feel in relationship to your partner? What is satisfying about this dance, and what feels limited?

Shift your movement exploration to initiate from the appendicular skeleton. How does this change the tone, the mood, and the quality of your relationship? What is satisfying about this dance, and what feels limited?

Take some time to explore a duet in which one partner initiates movement from the axial and the other partner from the appendicular skeleton. Shift roles, and notice how it changes the content, the quality, and the intention of your duet.

Finally, move together integrating the movement of your axial and appendicular skeletons. Notice how your habits emerge and what parts of your skeletal system tend to lead and which ones tend to follow.

Touch Explorations: Axial and Appendicular

Invite your partner to lie on their side. Slowly press into and gently move each of your partner's vertebral segments, from head to tail. Gently touch the bones of the cranium. Notice which levels of the axial skeleton move easily and feel resilient and vital. Notice if there are places that do not move or that seem to have restrictions.

Then have your partner lie supine. Map the bones of your partner's extremities—hands to shoulder girdle and ribs, feet to pelvic halves, and the bones of the face. Together with your partner, notice which bones of the appendicular skeleton feel active and alive and which feel quieter and less present.

Observation: Axial and Appendicular

Observe your partner moving. Notice whether movement tends to originate in the axis and flow to the limbs, whether it originates in the limbs and flow to the spine, or whether flow between axial and appendicular portions of the skeleton is limited.

Observe a variety of people in public spaces, noticing what preferences they display, which bones initiate their movement, and how each person's axial and appendicular skeletons express themselves differently.

Embodying Shafts and Joints

The long bones of the skeletal system have a common shape, varying primarily in size. Most long bones are located in the extremities, and include some of the largest bones of the body, such as the femur and humerus, as well as smaller ones such as the metacarpals and the phalanges.

A long bone is a shaft with two ends, each end forming part of a joint space. The shaft is the body of the bone, the part that creates shape and gives weight, length, and solidity. Moving from an embodied shaft provides a sense of power, stability, and weightedness, as well as an awareness of the architectural shape the body is expressing in space.

At each end of long bone is an articular surface that forms a joint with its neighboring bone, fitting together in various combinations of concavities and convexities: bases, heads, balls, and receptacles. The joints of most long bones are classified as diarthroses, or freely moveable joints. They are supported and guided by several different types of ligaments, which give the joint specificity, directionality, and stability. The articular spaces of the joints between long bones are filled with synovial fluid. Moving from an awareness of the joints, in contrast to the shafts, provides a sense of mobility, fluidity, sequencing, and directionality.

Movement Explorations: Shafts and Joints

Alone or with a partner, firmly touch the shafts of the bones of your arms and legs, allowing the bones to feel their depth, weight, and solidity. Initiate movement from the central portion of the bones, orienting your movement more toward stability. How does awareness of the shafts affect your weight, your movement with your partner, and your relationship to the environment?

Alone or with a partner, lightly touch all the joints along your arms and legs, inviting the joint spaces to feel fluid, open, and articulate. Initiate movement from your joints, and this time orient more toward mobility. How does awareness of the joints affect your weight, your movement with your partner, and your relationship to the environment? How is this experience different from initiating movement from the shafts of the bones?

Touching Shafts and Joints

With a partner lying on the floor, support one limb, holding and moving the shafts carefully in space. Make sure that the joints are respected and not strained, but sense the movement relating to the weight of the shafts.

Shift your touch to the joints. Hold them, allow them to move, and gently take each one through its range of motion. Feel movement arising from the slippery, gliding quality of the joints.

Embodying Synovial Fluid

Synovial is the fluid of free flow. It is a viscous liquid with the consistency of egg white produced and contained within the cavities of joints and the spaces between bursae and tendon sheaths. Embodiment of the slippery synovial fluid brings the qualities of looseness, relaxation, humor, and ease. It opens the joints, giving them an omni-directional potential, but also protects them by filling the joint space between the bones. Functionally, synovial fluid:

- Reduces friction and protects hyaline cartilage through lubrication

- Absorbs shock

- Supplies oxygen and nutrients to and removes carbon dioxide and metabolic wastes from the cells within articular cartilage

- Contains phagocytic cells that remove microbes and the debris that results from normal wear and tear in the joint.

The fluid-producing synovial membrane forms an inner layer within the joint cavity (Figure 3.2). The production of fluid, necessary for easy joint function, is stimulated by pressure and stretching of the synovial membrane. In the morning, when you stretch before getting out of bed, it is partly in order to wake up and stimulate your synovial fluid so that your joints will function easily. Any regular exercise will help to maintain the production of synovial fluid. If the fluid dries up or the synovial membranes do not release their liquids due to inflammatory processes, arthritis or other problems can emerge in the joint.

Embodied synovial fluid movement is indicative of how you inhabit your skeletal system. Some people

QR Code #2: Embodying Synovial Fluid

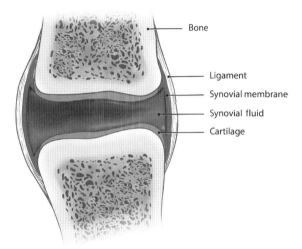

Figure 3.2

Synovial fluid in the joint

find a luxuriant rhythm of stretching and condensing, focused in the slipping and sliding sensation of deeply lubricated joints. Others find that the carefree, rebounding, unobstructed qualities of synovial fluid can be amusing, producing physical non-sequiturs and a goofy quality of loose-limbed play. However it emerges in your body, remember that the fluid itself is willing to go anywhere; it does not feel bound by the limitations of the joint structure. If you have a loose or injured joint make sure to take care of it during your explorations.

Finding Synovial Fluid

Making a gentle fist, move your wrist in flexion and extension. Feel the bones of your wrist moving against the bones of your forearm. What is your sensation?

Now visualize and feel the negative space between your bones, the joint space. Initiate movement not by moving the bones, but by changing the shape of the joint space. Sense how the shifting space between the bones changes the quality and tone of the movement. What is your sensation?

Finally visualize and feel the synovial fluid that fills the joint space of your wrist. Let the slippery quality of egg white mobilize the joint, rather than initiating from the bones or the joint space. Enjoy the movement and assess how it feels. What is your sensation?

Allow neighboring joints to become involved in the synovial movement, and allow that little dance to sequence through your entire body. Remember that your intervertebral and costovertebral joints are synovial, your jaw is synovial, and your sacroiliac joints are synovial. Each synovial joint is like a little pond with the potential for fluid movement.

Sensual Synovial

Lying on the floor, mobilize all of your joints through synovial fluid, emphasizing the easy stretching and condensing motions that will stimulate your synovial membranes to produce fluid. Balance your movement through the center of your joints, and enjoy the sequencing of movement from joint to joint. Allow your entire body to join the dance and take your time to explore what movement emerges.

Jovial Synovial

Warm up your joints with gentle jiggling, bouncing, and rebounding. Allow your movement to develop the illogical quality of a *non sequitur*. Don't plan your movement, but follow the limitless possibilities inherent in the slippery qualities of your joints. Your legs may go different directions, your arms may flail, and you may find sudden and unexpected pathways for moving up and down in space. Enjoy the ride and allow yourself to feel a little crazy, in a synovial way.

Support Precedes Movement

In the moving body, efficient movement arises from the changing relationship between a moving body part and the foundation of a stable body part. The stable part plays the role of support until it is time for the stable part to move, and then another part will take the support role. If the stable member does not yield into the earth as it supports the moving body part, then the movement will likely be constrained or inefficient. Several familiar words and phrases remind us of that principle: find your grounding, go down to go up, and ready, get set, go.

In the skeletal system, we need to constantly renew the flow of weight through our bones into the earth in order to move easily in space. Much of the work we do in somatic awareness is to find the most efficient pathway for movement, so that the flow of weight into the earth can be matched by the earth's force coming back into our bodies.

Support Precedes Movement Prone

Lying prone on the ground, release the weight of each bone into the earth. Remember that the earth is moving toward your body as your body is pouring into the earth. Push away from the earth starting with your hands, but as you do so listen to the quality of their connection with the earth: feel their width, their length, and the palms and fingers sitting on the earth as you move. Feel the support of your hands and forearms as your other bones continue to move away from the earth. Does this support make your movement easier?

Support Precedes Movement Standing

Move freely in space, but minimize your contact with the earth. Support with only a part of your foot, and do not release your weight into the ground. What is your experience? Then move or dance freely in space, but maximize your contact with the floor. Yield to the support of the earth as you move. How does your experience differ compared to the previous exploration?

Proximal and Distal

Proximal means toward the center of the body. Distal means away from the center of the body. The terms proximal and distal describe relationships, not places. In order for them to be useful in describing skeletal movement, we need to be clear about which bones and joints we are describing.

At any joint, there is a proximal bone (nearer to the center) and a distal bone (farther from the center). The femur is proximal to the tibia; the tibia is distal to the femur. The femur is distal to the pelvis; the pelvis is proximal to the femur.

In a general way, distal initiation indicates that movement is initiated from the extremity, such as the fingertips leading the arm and shoulder through space. Proximal initiation means that the movement starts near the core and radiates through a limb.

Proximal and Distal Movement

At any joint, distal movement occurs when the proximal bone is stabilized and the distal bone is free to move in space. Proximal movement occurs when the distal bone at a joint is stabilized as a support and the proximal bone moves (Hartley, 1995). At the elbow, moving the forearm with a fixed humerus is a distal movement (Figure 3.3); moving the humerus with a fixed forearm is a proximal movement (Figure 3.4). As a little test for yourself identify the proximal and distal bones at the following joints, and figure out how to perform distal and proximal movement at each one:

- The knee
- The ankle
- The wrist
- The jaw.

Finally, work on a problem that many students find difficult at first: find a way to perform proximal movement at the shoulder joint.

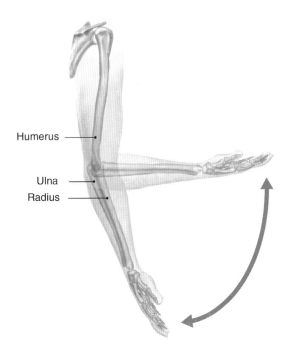

Figure 3.3

Distal movement at the elbow

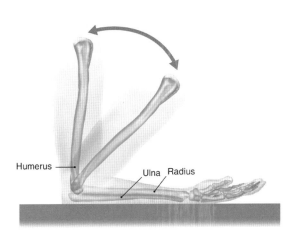

Figure 3.4

Proximal movement at the elbow

Equanimity in the Joints

In each joint there is a fluid-filled space cushioning the articulating bones. When the forces of weight and impact are consistently centered and flow evenly through a joint during weight bearing and movement, the joint remains untroubled. The word equanimity is derived from the Latin *aequanimitas* meaning "having an even mind." We want the mind of our joints to be even and undisturbed in movement, in order to preserve a sensation of balanced flow. The sensation of equanimity in the joint – which Bonnie Bainbridge Cohen calls "even and consistent joint space" – encourages effortlessness, resilience, an optimal range of movement, and minimal wear and tear on its internal structures (Bainbridge Cohen, 1997). When forces travel on a tangent to the axis of a joint, however, parts of that joint may become overly compressed or even immobile. Those unbalanced forces and habitual misalignments may result in overly tense or slack muscles, immobility or hypermobility in surrounding ligaments and fascia, nerve compression, and lack of circulation. The joint may eventually experience distress, pain, and diminishment of its movement—it will have lost its equanimity.

Most of the work we do with the bones and joints has the ultimate goal of establishing equanimity in the joints. Where one joint is free, it promotes ease of motion in its neighbors as well. The following ideas are important components of joint equanimity.

Centering the Weight

As the weight of the body flows through each joint, centering the weight within the joint will allow for equanimity.

Rotation and Traveling

In a ball-and-socket joint, the bone that forms the ball will rotate within the socket, if the socket is in the fixed bone (Figure 3.6). If the ball is fixed in space, the socket will travel over the ball (Figure 3.5). For instance, at the hip joint, the head of the femur rotates within the acetabulum when

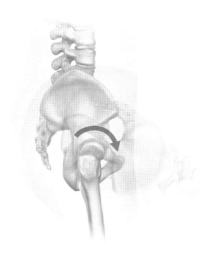

Figure 3.5

Traveling

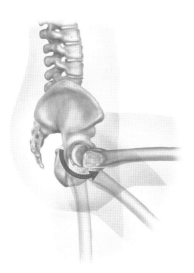

Figure 3.6

Rotation

the pelvis is fixed, such as in lying supine. If we flex at the hip joint when standing, the acetabulum will glide, traveling over the head of the femur.

Countermovement

From the perspective of the joint in motion, both bones are moving, although one may remain still in space. We can feel the movement of each bone countering the movement of the other.

Cogwheel Rotation

Cogwheel rotation is a combination of rotation, traveling, and countermovement. It is a useful principle to enhance equanimity when both bones at a joint are moving in space. Experiencing the combination of movements creates the sensation of mutual counter rotation of bones moving toward each other, just as two interconnected gears move in relationship to each other, each rotating in opposite directions.

Embodying the Three Layers of Bone (Figure 3.7)

Most of our bones consist of an outer membrane, the periosteum, that is continuous with the ligaments, tendons, and fascial matrix of the body; a dense mineralized portion, the compact bone, which provides strength and density; and a soft, flowing central core of marrow, a specialized fatty tissue that weds the skeletal system with our endocrine, immune, and blood production systems. Years ago I learned in classes with BMC^{SM} teacher Vera Orlock that as we embody and move through each layer of bone tissue, we invite sensations to arise that resonate through the entire body, providing body-mind states of expansion, solidity, and deep internal flow.

Periosteum

The outermost layer of bone, the periosteum, is a membrane surrounding the hard bone. Like paint covering a pencil, periosteum is the protective coating of our

QR Code #3: Moving from the Three Layers of Bone

Hard Bone: Compact and Spongy

Like the wood of a pencil, compact and spongy bone are the components of the mineral-rich hard bone, the middle layer that gives bone its shape and contour. While hard bone is the basis of what we recognize as the skeleton, it is important to remember that hard bone while alive contains fluids, living cells, and elastic components that give it flexibility and responsiveness.

Found in the shafts of long bones, compact bone is the densest and hardest part of the bone. It is specialized for the functions of protection and support, and allows our bones to resist gravity. Hard bone is the major reservoir of calcium in the body, needed for many metabolic processes.

Spongy bone, which is found at the ends of long bones and in irregularly shaped bones, has more space within it than does compact bone as well as a more generous blood supply. Spongy bone is arranged in a latticework, called trabeculae. Formed by the stresses placed on the bone, trabeculae shift and change as the forces moving through the bone are altered by new patterns of movement.

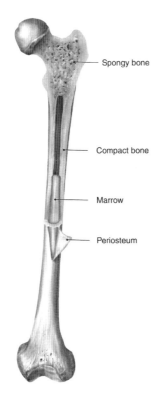

Spongy bone

Compact bone

Marrow

Periosteum

Figure 3.7

The three layers of bone

Marrow

The marrow is the viscous fluid layer at the center of the bone, corresponding to the central canal of graphite in a pencil. In adults, the cavity at the center of the shaft of the long bone (the medullary cavity) is inhabited by yellow marrow composed of fat. Red marrow is found in adults in the ends of the long bones (within the trabeculae of the spongy bone) and in flat bones, including the scapulae, sternum, ribs, and skull. Red marrow contains immature blood cells, fat, and cells of the immune system. It produces red blood cells, white blood cells, and platelets.

In the following explorations, trust your sensation and your imagination. With practice, we find that distinguishing the layers of bone becomes a reality, and is an important tool both for embodiment and repatterning movement.

bones. The outermost layer of periosteum is composed of dense, irregular connective tissue and is continuous with the ligaments and tendons that anchor themselves to it. It is rich with blood vessels, nerves, and lymphatic vessels that enter the bone. The inner layer of the periosteum is composed of elastic fibers and contains the osteoprogenitor cells that continually renew our bone. It is essential for the growth and repair of bone tissue. Observing and touching the glistening and slippery white surface of an uncooked chicken bone gives you a sense of your own human periosteum.

Movement Exploration: Three Layers of Bone

Alone or with a partner, stimulate the periosteum of all the bones of one limb with a very light touch that skims the surface of the bone. Allow the resonance of the touch to awaken the skin of your bone. Invite that sensation to initiate movement in space from the surface of the bone. Attend to the quality of movement that arises in the exploration and notice how initiating movement at the periosteum alters your mind—its quality of attention.

By yourself or with a partner, stimulate the hard bone with a firmer touch, not squeezing but allowing your awareness to descend into the hard bone. Allow the resonance of the touch to guide your bones into movement from the hard bone. Attend to the quality of movement that arises in the exploration and notice how your mind—its quality of attention—is altered by initiation of movement from the hard bone.

By yourself or with a partner, stimulate marrow with a deep and fluid touch. Imagine that you are holding a rain stick, feeling the seeds—the marrow—flowing within. Or that you are holding a stiff tube within which a thick liquid is moving slowly. Allow the resonance of the touch to guide your bones into movement from the marrow. Attend to the quality of movement that arises in the exploration and notice how your mind—its quality of attention—is altered by initiation of movement from the marrow.

Three Layers of Bone in a Pencil

Sitting comfortably, place a pencil between your thumbs and fingers and imagine transforming it into a living bone.

Feel the skin-like painted surface of the pencil. Imagine it as a resilient living substance like periosteum.

Allow the sensation in your fingers to drop deeply into the pencil and connect with the hard wood beneath the paint—the hard bone. Try shifting your attention back and forth between the feeling of the surface (periosteum) and the feeling of the wood (hard bone) underneath.

Allow the sensation in your fingers to feel more deeply into the soft center of the pencil, the graphite. It is like the marrow.

Feel the presence of paint, wood, and lead together and separately.

Touching the Three Layers of Bone

Sitting comfortably with a partner, share a moment of breathing together. Become aware of your own skin. When you feel embodied in your own skin, place your hands on your partner's forearm, and feel for this same quality of surface in your partner. Drop your awareness to the layer of muscles underneath your own skin. Feel for the resonance of that quality in your partner's muscles. That does not mean increasing the pressure, although it can mean shifting how you experience the weight of your hand, and it can mean a different quality of touch. Feel how the mood, the mind, shifts for both of you.

Drop your awareness underneath the layer of muscle to the periosteum of your forearm bones. Feel for the resonance of that layer in your partner's body. The periosteum can feel floaty or expansive. It can have a nervous quality. It can feel tight and constricted or loose and easygoing. It may be comfortable or uncomfortable to sense. You may want to slide the surrounding fascia and skin over the periosteum, shining it up!

In your own body, drop your awareness deeper, to the hard bone. Feel for the resonance of that new layer in your partner's body. Feel how the mood shifts in both you and your partner. The hard bone often brings a deepened quality of presence—"I am here"—and may invite skeletal adjustments in the entire body.

Finally, drop your awareness to the marrow at the core of your bone. Feel for the resonance of marrow in your partner's body. Feel how the mind shifts in both you and your partner. The marrow often brings a sense of flow, like a streamlet at the center of the bone, or it can feel sluggish and stale. The marrow often encourages a sense of relationship to neighboring bones, as though the stream flows from bone to bone.

When finished, ask your partner to compare the sensation in that forearm with the sensation in the arm you have not touched. Share your experience with each other.

The Elements of Skeletal Touch

Conscious touch can support self-awareness in any tissue, which creates the possibility for movement. We use touch in the skeletal system to bring awareness to bone, to support self-healing processes within the bone, and to repattern inefficient movement habits toward ones that support easier bone and joint function. Most techniques of communicating with bone through touch can be applied to almost any bone or joint in the body. They include bone mapping, releasing bone from myofascial binding, and joint compression and release. When you have mastered these basic elements of skeletal touch they will begin to blend together in your work, and become a continuous fabric of expression, interwoven with each other in your play with bones. It is always helpful to return to the basics, and practice each touch or skill individually, as described below.

Bone Mapping

Bone mapping is an easy way to bring self-awareness to individual bones and to the skeletal structure as a whole. By outlining the contours of each bone with touch, you create a sensory map of the skeletal system that helps to individuate bones from flesh and surrounding tissues. Called "bone tracing" by Bonnie Bainbridge Cohen, mapping bones is much like using a yellow highlighter to identify the essence of a text, allowing you to return to the passage at a later date. Having highlighted the bones, they remain available for efficient and consistently pleasurable movement.

Exploration of Bone Mapping

When mapping the skeletal structure, we are particularly concerned with enlivening the periosteum. Here is a simple approach to mapping the bones of one finger. The same procedure can be applied to any other bone.

With the fingers of one hand, gently and sensitively feel through the flesh of the tip (distal phalanx) of the index finger of the opposite hand, until your awareness lands on the surface of the bone. Don't squeeze: try to land gently on the surface. Walk your active fingers around its contours waking up the surface of the bone and try a little gliding and sliding to stimulate the periosteum.

Repeat the exploration for each bone of the index finger. When you finish this process, notice what the sensation of the finger is compared with the sensation of your other fingers.

Do the same with a partner's bones—a finger, an arm, or the entire body—and discuss the resulting sensations. Some suggestions for bone mapping:

- Map all the bones of your partner's arm. When finished, ask them to compare the sensation in the arm that was mapped with that of the other arm. Is it heavy? Light? Tingly? Aware? Alive?

- Map the bones of your partner's entire body. You can do bone mapping in detail or relatively quickly, as a warm up for other explorations or as a preparation for movement. Share feedback when finished.

Releasing Bone from Myofascial Binding

Areas of our bodies, such as our forelegs, can be experienced as masses without distinct internal parts. If muscle and the supporting fascia are trying to do the work of bone, rather than being used to simply move the bones, then the bone underlying those overactive muscles may not recognize its own capacities and functions. The result is that the body part is experienced as an undifferentiated unit, instead of a balanced composition of its parts, each with a different function. Like bone mapping, releasing bone from myofascial binding develops the individuated awareness of bone.

Exploration of Releasing Bone

With a partner lying on the floor, stabilize the bones of one limb with your hand. Grasping the overlying muscle in the other, slide the flesh horizontally around the bone, gently at first and then feeling for deeper and deeper mobility of the flesh. Finally, you should be able to free the meeting place between the muscle and bone. Shift your hands as needed to access each part of the limb. Be aware of

working deeply in the center of the muscle bellies and more sensitively around the joints.

Check in frequently with your partner to make sure that what you're doing feels comfortable. When finished with one limb, ask them to compare the sensation between finished and unfinished limbs. Repeat with the other limbs.

Joint Compression and Release

Each joint of a long bone has a ligamentous joint capsule, enclosing a fluid space. With age and various forms of stress, the joint can lose its equanimity and the fluid content will be diminished. Gentle joint compression and release can encourage joints to return to optimal function. Compression stimulates the production of synovial fluid and provides proprioceptive self-awareness within the joint. The release supports resilience and the internal space. The technique of compression and release stimulates the joint proprioceptors and supports both mobility and stability within the joint.

Exploration of Joint Compression and Release

Identify any joint in your partner's body. Gently grasp the bones on each side of that joint and simply notice the relationship between the two bones. Bring the ends of the bones together until they meet: introduce them to each other as if for the first time. Wait for a sense of rebound or expansion within the joint, and follow the movement of the bones as they open away from the joint. Notice if the relationship between the bones has been altered and whether there is a different sensation. Try doing the same with a number of joints and discuss with your partner how their body feels as a result of the exploration.

Levering Through the Bones

Levering is the use of joint compression to track the flow of information through the skeletal system from one bone to the next. Levering is generally initiated from distal bones toward the core—for instance, from ankle to knee to hip to sacroiliac. Specific levering explorations are described in other chapters.

Breath, Vibration, and Sound

Living bone benefits from and responds to the stimulation of conscious breathing and the vibration of sound. Both responses occur on the cellular level of organization rather than the tissue level. They are tools that can be used to support transformation and awareness within ourselves or in other people.

Cellular Respiration in Bone

The cell is the fundamental unit of self-replicating life. As humans, we have about 70 trillion cells within our bodies that are genetically identified as belonging to ourselves, and we are hosts as well to many other cells belonging to the microbiome. Our health depends on the individual health and well being of each cell in our bodies. As animals descended from single-celled organisms, we are composed of vast colonies of specialized cells. Where there is restriction or confusion in a cell or group of cells within the skeleton, that stress can ultimately contribute to disease or chronic dysfunction. Increasing ease at a cellular level contributes directly to general health—in this case to skeletal health—and to the body's natural recuperative abilities. We can do that by inviting breath into each cell of the skeleton, through meditation on cellular respiration, and through improving skeletal alignment and habits of movement to create space for cellular respiration.

Cellular respiration—the constant expanding and condensing motion of breath—is the movement constellation of one-celled animals and all cells within us. External respiration, the familiar breathing of the chest, lungs, and nasal passageway, exhibits

QR Code #4: Cellular Respiration in Bone

the same oscillation of expanding and condensing space. External respiration occurs in service of internal respiration, providing oxygen to every cell.

To explore the movement of cellular respiration you do not need to work with the immense complexity of the cell, but very simply with its three major elements: the internal fluid world, the external fluid world, and the membrane that separates those two worlds. The environment for cellular breath is water, both in the single-celled creatures of the prehistoric ocean and in our own multicellular beings. Our cells thrive in a fluid medium called the interstitial fluid, a version of the early sea within our bodies, as much in bone as in our other tissues. Water is also the primary constituent of the cytosol, the internal ocean of the cell.

Cellular Respiration in Bone

Find a comfortable resting position. Observe your lungs filling and emptying as you breathe. Release any tension you might find in your diaphragm, chest, and neck, so as to allow three-dimensional movement in your chest and lungs.

Imagine that your skin is the membrane of a large cell and that everything inside your skin is fluid. Allow your three-dimensional skin to expand outwardly as you breathe in and to release toward your center as you exhale. Imagine that you are drifting in a fluid environment, supported by water and composed of water, separated by skin, your expanding and condensing membrane. During the exploration you may find yourself deepening into relaxation, slowing down your mental processes, and becoming more aware of the present moment.

If you wish to go farther, you can imagine or feel within yourself the presence of an individual cell or a small group of cells within your bone structure. Just as you experienced expanding and condensing movement in your entire body, you can sense the expanding and condensing breath of individual cells. Feel them expanding and condensing, floating, and breathing. Spread the sensation to your entire skeleton. Allow your cells to initiate your external respiration, as though they are the roots of breath deep within you. Notice what changes occur in your consciousness and in your body as you explore cellular respiration in your bones.

Cellular Touch

Touching another person with the resonance of cellular respiration is a non-invasive invitation to change. The touch encourages a partner's bone cells to find ease, to recuperate, and to make the adjustments necessary for health and optimal function.

Cellular Touch in Bone

Find a comfortable position, and make sure your partner is comfortable. Agree with your partner where you will provide cellular touch. Before you touch your partner:

1. Invite awareness of the expanding and condensing rhythm of breath in your own lungs. Pay attention to the three-dimensionality of breathing. Allow this awareness to flow into the other cavities of your torso and the head.

2. Allow the expanding and condensing rhythm to travel into your extremities. Feel spaciousness in time, and eliminate any sense of doing in favor of a sense of being. Allow an eternal beingness to permeate your breathing.

3. Bring awareness to the expanding and condensing of each cell in your body, not from the consciousness of the brain, but from the awareness of the cells themselves.

After your preparation:

Place your hands gently on your partner, not to do anything, but simply to be, your hands breathing next to and with your partner's body. Observe the breathing of the cells in your own bones, and feel for the resonance of cellular respiration expanding and condensing in your partner's bones. Float in this breath with your partner as long as you are able to maintain a sense of non-doing.

As you finish, compare you experiences with your partner—what you felt, what they felt, what changes may have occurred, and how your relationship changed during the exploration.

Sounding into Bone

Experientially, we know that sound is a powerful stimulus, with the potential to incite both alarm and relaxation in the nervous system. Sound affects us at a cellular level as well. The molecular structure of bone seems to respond to direct vibrational stimulus as well as to cellular touch. We can use our voices to transmit the information contained in vibration to various tissues, including bone, which may respond with a sense of pleasure and a stronger sense of self as a result.

Sounding into Bone

With a partner, use a steady breath to hum a soft, sustained tone, feeling the vibration in your voice and letting it resonate in surrounding tissues. Place your mouth on or near your partner's forearm, and let the vibration of sound enter through the skin and muscles into the bone.

Vary the pitch and the intensity of your voice. A softer sound can often penetrate more deeply. (Less is more!) You will feel when you have found the right pitch and intensity for the bone. It will resonate and vibrate freely with your voice.

Make a "zzzz" vibration between your front teeth, and project that sound into the bone. If either you or your partner is uncomfortable with the mouth-to-skin contact, place your fingers between your mouth and your partner's arm: make the "zzzz" sound into your own finger bones, and allow the bones to transmit the vibration into your partner. Work up and down your partner's bone. Note differences in the response at different sites. Ask your partner to compare the sensation in that arm with the arm that has not received the vibration.

Repeat with any bone, and enjoy.

The Lower Extremities

Embodying the Foot

Oh the foot, the amazing foot! We take it for granted most of the time, as it performs numerous tasks for us, paying attention to it only when it sends signals of distress. When cared for, the foot is a structural marvel: strong, light, adaptable, dependable, and mobile, receiving weight and stresses on a daily basis that are compounded greatly when we jump and run. If neglected or maltreated, it may complain loudly. The foot has many ways of giving us feedback about our movement habits, both the positive ones and the neglectful.

It has been said that we can repattern the entire body through the feet. That is because the tissues of the feet must respond and adapt to the movement choices we make higher in the body. Changing a building's foundation will necessarily change the shape of the structure on top of it, and so it is with our feet. They are the foundation of our moving bodies. So let's give a little prayer of thanks to our feet. The process of embodying them through bone will make them happy and support ease of movement through the legs and trunk.

Before we address the details of the skeletal foot, consider the present condition of your feet. What is their history? What have they supported you in doing: dancing, running, kicking, making love? Have they sustained breaks? Warts? Pain? Bunions? Hammertoes? What might you say are the characteristics of your feet? Which foot is dominant? If they had voices, what might they say to you? Do you

hide them, or make judgments about their appearance? I often think of my feet as little animals, with desires, understanding, and knowledge that I could learn from if I would just take the time to listen.

Cellular Respiration

Bring your awareness first to your own cellular respiration, emphasizing your bones. When your own breathing is well established, touch your partner's foot, maintaining awareness of the underlying skeletal structure. Allow your awareness to drop into the bone tissue: your pressure or tone might increase slightly in order to feel the skeletal presence, but the emphasis is on the cellular respiration of the bones, not on their structure. If movement arises within the tissue, follow the movement. If the foot remains resting, just enjoy the contact.

The Bones of the Foot (Figure 4.1)

Get to know the bones of your feet. They are like family members whose names you will always remember because they are part of your life.

The Phalanges

The phalanges are the bones of the toes. (A single bone is called a phalanx.) The big toe has two phalanges, distal and proximal, while the remaining four toes each have three: distal, middle and proximal. Joints between the phalanges are called interphalangeal joints, which move in flexion and extension. Each phalanx has a slightly concave base, a shaft, and a rounded head.

The Metatarsals

The five bones of the forefoot are called metatarsals. Each toe is supported by a metatarsal bone, with a base, a shaft, and a head. The first (big toe) metatarsal is the shortest and the thickest, and the fifth metatarsal has a palpable tuberosity on the lateral side of the foot. The articulations between the phalanges and the metatarsals are the metatarsophalangeal joints, which move in flexion/extension and abduction/adduction. The base of each metatarsal bone forms a joint with the tarsal bones, the tarsometatarsal joints, which move in flexion/extension and abduction/adduction. The heads of the metatarsals form a unit, joined by a transverse ligament. The bases of the metatarsals create a similar unit, formed by the intermetatarsal joints.

Fingers and Toes

To support mobility and individuation of the toes, interlace the toes of one foot with the fingers of the opposite hand. Move the toes gently and fluidly, and enjoy the contact of hand to foot. Finding space for your fingers may be difficult at first, but eventually the space in the forefoot will open, the metatarsal bones will widen and spread, and movement will be easier and more spacious.

The Tarsal Bones

The tarsals (the three cuneiforms and the navicular, cuboid, talus, and calcaneus) are the seven bones of the hindfoot. As a group, they allow the motions of flexion/extension, abduction/adduction, and rotation, permitting both pronation and supination.

Dorsal view

Plantar view

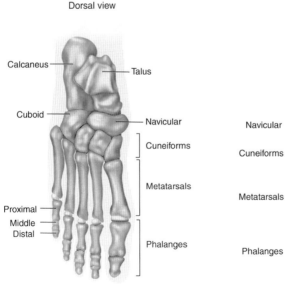
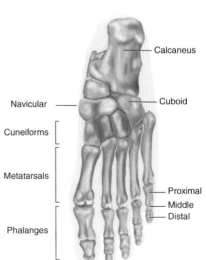

Figure 4.1

Bones of the foot, dorsal and plantar views

Cuneiforms

Cuneiform means wedge-shaped, and the three cunei-form bones—medial, intermediate, and lateral—form a tight arch over the medial side of the instep of the foot. They are situated between the metatarsals of the first three toes and the navicular bone, which receives the proximal surfaces of all three cunei-forms. The distal joints of the cuneiforms with the metatarsal bones are called the tarsometatarsals. The joints between the cuneiforms are called the intercu-neiform articulations. The joint between the lateral cuneiform and the cuboid bone is the cuneocuboid, and the articulations between the three cuneiforms and the navicular are the cuneonavicular joints.

Navicular

The boat-shaped navicular bone transmits forces between the cuneiforms and the talus. The tuberosity of the navicular is palpable in most people as a small bump on the medial side of the foot below and ante-rior to the medial malleolus. The articulation with the talus is the talonavicular joint.

Cuboid

Forming the lateral surface of the foot underneath the ankle, the cuboid bone transmits the lines of force between the fourth and fifth metatarsal bones and the calcaneus. Between the cuboid and the met-atarsals are the tarsometatarsal joints. The joint with the calcaneus is called the calcaneocuboid. There is also a joint between the cuboid and navicular bones.

Talus

The talus receives the weight of the entire body from the tibia, and spreads the forces it receives into the foot. It is a unique bone, having no muscular attach-ments. It is free-floating and responds to the forces of weight and ligamentous attachments with neigh-boring bones. It articulates with the tibia, the calca-neus, and the navicular bones.

Calcaneus

The calcaneus—the heelbone—is the largest of the tarsal bones. On its anterior surface is the joint with

the cuboid bone, the calcaneocuboid, which helps to form the lateral longitudinal arch of the foot. On its superior surface is the joint with the talus, the subtalar joint. The subtalar is a key joint in the ankle. It has three surfaces of articulation with three separate facet joints, which allow movement in each plane as well as pronation and supination. Part of the movement of the ankle happens in this joint; the rest occurs at the talar-tibial joint.

The bony unit of talus and navicular, with its tal-onavicular joint and the unit formed by the cal-caneus and the cuboid, with its calcaneocuboid joint, together form a compound joint, the trans-verse tarsal joint.

Freeing Articulations

Each bone in the foot has a joint with at least one other bone, and many have multiple articulations. Working through the foot, move the more flexible joints softly through their full range of motion. For the joints between the closely packed tarsal bones, identify the joints and find where there is gliding movement and where it is more restricted.

At joints that feel tight, you may want to try using less pressure or cellular touch to facilitate awareness.

The Rays of the Foot

Each toe is the product of a sequence of bones, a ray traveling deep into the mid-foot. Distal phalan-ges articulate in sequence with middle and proxi-mal phalanges, which connect with their respective metatarsals, and ultimately into tarsal bones along the same line. That arrangement creates radiating lines of force that connect each toe with a specific part of the hindfoot.

Mapping the Rays of the Foot

Use bone mapping as described in Chapter Three to create a sensory image of the rays of a partner's foot. Begin by mapping the distal phalanx of the big toe. Sequence through the proximal phalanx and the first metatarsal to the joint with the first cuneiform and finally into the navicular. Repeat with each toe, encouraging the foot to feel its longitudinal organization. The fourth and fifth toes both lead into the cuboid bone.

Invite your partner to stand and observe the difference in sensation between the foot that has been mapped and the foot that was not. Are there changes of sensation or position in the foot or in any other part of the body? Invite your partner to walk from the felt sense of the bones in the foot. Repeat the mapping on the other foot.

Grounding Through the Foot

In standing, walking, and running, our feet communicate with the earth. They can alert us to patterns of weight falling through the body, so listening to them is an important sensory tool for alignment. Ideally, the entire surface of the foot is sensate, and weight is distributed evenly throughout.

If weight is placed habitually forward or back on the foot, compensation is required in muscle, ligament, and tendon, preventing a free flow of weight through the body. If weight is centered in the middle of the ankle joint and distributed through the whole foot, the body is free to release the extra work needed to support verticality. You can live more responsively and creatively in the present moment.

Grounding Through the Foot: Standing

In order to assess your relationship with the earth, stand for a moment and determine whether your weight falls more through your heels, more through the front of your foot, or through the talus with an evenly distributed flow of weight to the whole foot. Rock gently, initiating from your pelvis and your whole trunk. Feeling the soles of your feet on the floor, sense the shifting pressure as your weight eases from back to front, side to side, and in looping improvised patterns.

Feel where in your body you need to compensate muscularly as you move in each direction. Which joints and surfaces tighten? Which ones relax? For instance, shift your weight to the front and notice what happens to your calves, thighs, lower back, and shoulders. What happens at the same time in the front of your body?

Allow the motion to get smaller and smaller until you reach a point where you stop, but the swaying is still occurring at an energetic or microscopic level. Can you come to rest in a place where the talus is situated directly under your sitting bones? Are the back and front of your body both released? Can your head and neck rise effortlessly toward the sky?

Grounding Through the Foot: Making Pancakes

Imagine pancake batter being poured onto a griddle, and observe how it spreads evenly from the center in every direction. Then feel your weight pouring through your lower legs. When it arrives in your feet, allow it to spread evenly in every direction on the floor, like batter on the griddle. Permit your feet to spread and take up more space on the floor.

Experiment with small steps. Each time you put a foot on the earth, allow the pancake batter to spread and use it to relax your feet completely.

Grounding Through the Foot: Walking

First bring your awareness to the flow of your breath, and the sensation of your foot on the floor. As you begin walking, notice how and where your foot strikes the ground. What is the sequence of contact?

Emphasize weight falling through your heel. What does that do to the sensation in your ankle and in your whole body?

Emphasize weight falling in your forefoot. How does that change the sensation in your ankle and body?

Experiment with utilizing your whole foot, feeling the stride rocking through from back to front, with your weight centered in the talus. How does the shift in emphasis change the sensations in your ankle, foot, and body?

Mobile Foot and Stable Foot

If a bridge is too stiff, it will be brittle and fail as environmental forces such as wind, earthquakes, and water act upon it. If it is built with too much pliancy, it will not be able to bear the weight it is meant to carry. Our feet need to be equally responsive to the contradictory demands of stability and mobility.

Nature has provided an elegant solution to address those contradictory needs. There are two separate skeletal units within each foot, one—the stable foot—that serves the needs of stability, and another that serves the needs of mobility, the mobile foot (Figure 4.2). The stable foot is lateral, extending from the calcaneus to the fourth and fifth toes. The mobile foot is medial, extending from the talus through the navicular into the first three rays of toes (Bainbridge Cohen, 1995, pp. 2–3). The mobile foot possesses more bones than the stable foot: where there are more bones, there are more articulations, and where there are more articulations, there is more mobility (Table 4.1). If seen from above or from below, a clear division somewhat like a clamshell opening is evident in the tarsal area between the stable foot and the mobile foot.

When weight flows through the foot in a balanced way, there are clear distinctions between these two functional units:

- When we are standing, the force of weight pours from the leg through the talus onto the calcaneus and is distributed forward and backward through the lateral longitudinal arch of the foot. This is the stable foot.

- When we are pushing away from the earth in walking, running, or rising onto our toes, the primary pathway of force shifts, following a line from the rays of the first three toes through the cuneiforms, the navicular, the talus, and into the leg. This is the mobile foot.

In standing, the primary line of force is the downward flow from the tibia into the stable foot; the upward counterflow of the mobile foot is secondary. When we are moving, the primary line of force is the upward flow through the mobile foot; the downward counterflow of the stable foot is secondary.

Confusion in using the stable foot and the mobile foot creates serious issues within the foot, including postural pronation, supination, bunions, and hammertoes. It can also reflect into different parts of the body, with pain at the knee, hip, sacroiliac joints or the lower back.

Pronation and Supination of the Foot

Pronation and supination are natural and necessary movements of the foot, ankle, and lower legs that adapt the body to moving on uneven terrain. They allow the

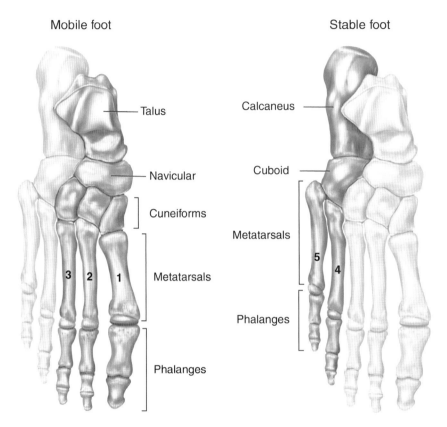

Figure 4.2

Mobile foot and stable foot

Table 4.1: Bones of the Mobile Foot and Stable Foot

Bones of the Mobile Foot	Bones of the Stable Foot
Phalanges of the first three toes	Phalanges of the fourth and fifth toes
First three metatarsals	Fourth and fifth metatarsals
Cuneiforms	Cuboid
Navicular	Calcaneus
Talus	

feet to accommodate to small tilts, bumps, and objects without destabilizing the whole skeletal structure. Life indoors, constant walking on flat pavement, and the continual wearing of shoes diminish the need to utilize our feet in this adaptive way. Lacking that natural stimulation, our feet can get stuck in the expression of pronation or supination, and the resulting immobility demands compensations that refer discomfort or dysfunction to the legs, pelvis, or back.

Pronation and supination are complex movements that involve actions at many joints. Each involves movement through three planes: sagittal, vertical, and horizontal. There is a specialized vocabulary to describe the movement of the foot in the planes:

Sagittal Plane

Sagittal plane motion is called dorsiflexion when the toes move toward the knees and plantar flexion when the toes move away from the knees. The articulations that support these movements are the tibio-talar and subtalar joints.

Vertical Plane

Vertical plane motion is called adduction when the sole of the foot moves toward the midline, and abduction when the sole of the foot moves away from midline. The joints that support adduction and abduction are the subtalar and transverse talar joints.

Horizontal Plane

The movement of the horizontal plane is rotation. In the ankle and foot, external rotation—when the sole of the foot moves outward, away from midline— is termed eversion. Inversion occurs when the sole of the foot moves medially, toward or past midline. The joints that support eversion and inversion are the subtalar, transverse talar, tarsometatarsal joints and joints between the tibia and fibula. Eversion is sometimes thought to be the same as pronation and inversion synonymous with supination. In fact, eversion is a component of pronation and inversion a component of supination.

When we analyze the movement of pronation we see that it combines subtalar eversion, ankle dorsiflexion, and forefoot abduction. In a fixed position, pronation favors weight-flow through the mobile foot, which collapses the medial longitudinal arch of the foot, while the medial malleolus of the tibia moves toward midline of the body.

Supination is a combination of subtalar inversion, plantar flexion of the ankle, and forefoot adduction. If supination becomes a habit in weight bearing, it creates an emphasis on the stable foot, the lateral surface of the foot, and it lifts the medial longitudinal arch excessively. The lateral malleolus of the fibula may move away from the midline of the body.

Mobile Foot and Stable Foot: Standing and Walking

Feel and observe the habits of your feet in standing. Does each foot receive the weight of your body evenly? Are they more expressive of mobile foot or of stable foot? Is there a tendency toward pronation or toward supination?

Are your feet the same, or do you perceive different patterns of weight flow between them? Can you bring awareness to all the bones of your feet equally?

Experiment with the same questions in walking.

Observe the habits of others in standing and walking. How do they utilize their mobile feet and their stable feet?

Neutral Alignment

A plumb line is a string with a weight at one end that builders use to provide a vertical reference line. To align weight systematically through the skeletal system, we can map the most efficient pathway for weight flow by visualizing a plumb line falling through specific points in our bones.

The reference point for optimal alignment is anatomical position. In standing, this is with the feet in parallel planted directly beneath the hip joints rather than below the iliac crests or wider, and knees and toes directed forward. In that stance a plumb line for each leg falls from the center of the hip joint through the ray of the second toe, passing through the intercondylar space at the center of the knee and the center point of the ankle. (See Figure 5.1, page 84.)

Mobile Foot/Stable Foot: Standing Alignment

The pronation/supination patterns in the foot are often established in relation to movement habits originating in higher joints: the sacroiliac, hips, or knees. Standing in front of a mirror, observe the alignment of your hip joints, knees, and ankles. Note whether the knees and ankles are wider than the centers of your hip joints. Is there a plumb line falling through the center of your hip joint to the center of your knee to the center of your ankle? Note whether the toes and knees seem to be pointing forward toward the mirror or if they are rotated in an inward or outward direction.

If your joints do not fall into a plumb line beneath you, see what happens to the relationship between your mobile foot and your stable foot if you adjust your stance so that the centers of your hips, knees, and ankles fall into alignment. If one or more joints seem to be rotating in inward or outward, see what happens to the relationship between your mobile foot and your stable foot when you direct the knee and the toes forward in space.

What happens to the relationship between your mobile foot and stable foot when you fold simultaneously at the ankle, knee, and hip joints? How does the change that occurs relate to the inward or outward motion of your knees through space as they bend?

Dividing Mobile Foot and Stable Foot

Help your partner to sense the division between the stable foot and mobile foot. Hold the heads of your partner's fourth and fifth metatarsals in one hand and first through third metatarsals with your other hand. Gently move the two groups of metatarsals in opposite directions, up and down, stretching the fascia and ligaments that bind the third and fourth metatarsals.

Progress longitudinally along the bones, simultaneously moving one up and one down to free the tissue between the bones. Continue this alternating pattern through the length of the metatarsals.

Ask your partner how it feels and invite them to stand and register any changes.

Movement at the Subtalar Joint

The subtalar joint between the talus and the calcaneus is the point of transition between the mobile foot and the stable foot when the foot is in motion. Where there is confusion between mobility and stability in the ankle and foot, releasing that joint can be the key to providing clarity.

Moving the Subtalar Joint

By holding your own calcaneus (with a gentle embrace of the heel) and the talus (just under the medial and lateral malleoli), you can feel the movement in the joint and ask the joint what it wants to do. Remember that there is potential for movement in each of the three planes. Follow the movement if you perceive any.

Embodying the Ankle Joint

The ankle is formed by three bones, the tibia, the fibula, and the talus, and is the point of articulation between the foreleg and the foot (Figure 4.3). The tibia and the fibula form a malleolar mortise, with a concave receptacle at the distal end of the tibia to fit the curvature of the talus. The joint surface of the fibula extends further distally than does the tibia. The primary motions at the ankle joint are plantar flexion and dorsiflexion. Its secondary motions are inversion and eversion.

In its primary motion of plantar and dorsiflexion, the ankle joint does not function as a hinge, as most people imagine. Rather, the tibia slides over the arc of the talus in a gliding, curving pathway. When the ankle is embodied, awareness of that sliding action can increase range of motion in the joint and contribute to pliant and resilient functioning of the feet. In my history as a dance student, I was often told to "point your toes," which was intended as a cue to plantar-flex at the ankle joint. As a result of that instruction, I tried to initiate the movement with my toes for many years, and couldn't understand why my ankle felt so locked. Finally, I learned that the movement can be initiated by sliding the talus underneath the tibia. Gradually my ankle became free and juicy, and I was able to increase my range of motion (Figure 4.4).

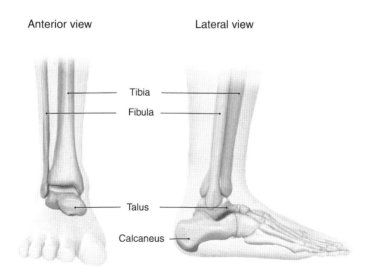

Anterior view   Lateral view

Tibia

Fibula

Talus

Calcaneus

Right ankle joint

Figure 4.3

The ankle joint

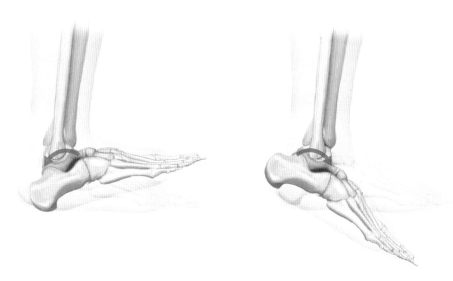

Figure 4.4

Sliding in the ankle joint

Sliding the Ankle

Sit in such a way that your foot is free in space, the ankle available for distal movement. Initiate plantar flexion and dorsiflexion inside the ankle joint rather than with the toes, thinking of a water wheel turning in the sagittal plane between the malleoli as you move. Feel the rounded arc of the talus rotate within the convex tibial surface and enjoy the fluid viscosity of the joint. Let the rest of your foot respond to that internal motion, allowing your toes to hang free and take a ride. When you dorsiflex, feel the heel reaching diagonally backward and downward in space from the ankle joint. Imagine eyes on the back of the talus peeking out in the open space just below the tibia. In plantar flexion, feel the tarsals sliding toward the front in a forward and downward diagonal. Imagine eyes on the talus peeking out in front, below the tibia.

In standing, fold and unfold the leg at the ankle, knee, and hip joints, initiating from the fluid sensation of the tibia gliding over the talus.

Sliding a Partner's Ankle

This exploration helps your partner to embody the slippery quality of the ankle joint. It is especially helpful for people with limitation in the joint. Position your partner in such a way that the foot is free in space, the knee is slightly bent, and you have access to the foot with both hands. You may have to rest your partner's leg on your own thigh.

Place one hand on your partner's calcaneus and the other on the forefoot. Mentally map the arc of the talus underlying the tibia, and then begin to encourage movement along that arc. Use your hands so the talus and calcaneus travel through space in an arcing pathway, diagonally posterior and inferior, taking the foot into dorsiflexion. That should feel more spacious in the joint than pushing the heel directly down to dorsiflex.

Find the gliding pathway into plantar flexion. Use your hands to guide the talus and navicular bones in an arc, diagonally anterior and inferior, taking the foot into plantar flexion. That should feel more spacious than pushing the toes down into plantar flexion.

Repeat those motions several times, and encourage the joint to feel relaxed, lubricated, and spacious. How does that affect the sensation in the ankle? Invite your partner to stand and walk, and compare the sensation of that ankle with the other.

Proximal Origination for Distal Movement and Distal Origination for Proximal Movement

When movement is preceded by support in a joint, it means that there is awareness in the supporting bone as the moving bone shifts in space. Whichever bone is in the support role, whether distal or proximal, we can focus on the articular surface of that bone for the origination of the movement, even though the other bone will be seen to be moving. When we do that, the quality of movement changes. Less effort is required, alignment improves, and there is equanimity within the joint space.

Think of a movement at any joint. Imagine that the joint surface of the supporting bone is covered with a plush velvet cloth. When you decide to move, first change the nap of the velvet of the supporting bone in the direction of the movement, and continue to feel the surface of the support bone as the moving bone shifts in space.

Having experienced sliding in the ankle joint, you can use this idea to bring even greater specificity to the origination of ankle movement. At the ankle, the distal bone is the talus, and the tibia is proximal. If you originate movement clearly from awareness in the support bone, whether proximal or distal, the moving bone will slide more freely through its range of motion. The explorations below provide several ways to find support at the ankle prior to moving.

Distal and Proximal Origination in the Ankle

Proximal Origination for Distal Movement

Sitting or lying down, with the foot free in space, visualize and feel the concave joint surface of the tibia. Imagine that concave surface covered with velvet.

Before moving the ankle, imagine that the nap of the velvet on the tibia will shift in the direction of the intended movement. When that image is strong in your felt sense, allow the talus to respond by rotating, sliding along the articular surface, moving into plantar flexion or dorsiflexion. How does that change your experience of moving the ankle?

Distal Origination of Proximal Movement

Standing, feel the rounded joint surface of the talus rising toward the supporting surface of the tibia, and sense its form. Imagine the articular surface of the talus covered with velvet. Before bending the ankle to make a small plié, imagine that the nap of the velvet will shift in the direction of the intended movement. When that image is strong in your felt sense, allow the tibia to respond to the invitation of the velvety talus by traveling over the rounded surface. How does that change your experience of moving the leg at the ankle? How does that change your experience in the other joints above it?

Embodying the Foreleg

The lower leg is a passageway for weight, funneling the combined forces of the upper body into the earth. It also plays a part in refining the movements of our knees and ankles.

We may take the foot for granted, but the frequency with which we forget or overlook the foreleg is absolutely unfair given its functions. If we do not acknowledge the complexity and the dynamic movement that is intrinsic to its structure, an unembodied lower leg can feel wooden and undifferentiated. Get to know your bones and distinguish their functions, so that you experience the foreleg not as an undifferentiated mass but as an articulate pathway that connects knee with ankle.

Releasing the Foreleg from Myofascial Binding

Because the foreleg is often experienced as a single discreet mass, lacking discrimination among its parts, it is helpful to provide an experience of individuated awareness of bone separate from the awareness of muscle. Follow the suggestions in Chapter 3 for releasing bone from binding, working with your partner's muscle and fascia surrounding the tibia and fibula. Feel for changes in tone, vitality, and resilience. When you have finished, invite your partner to move the foreleg, initiating movement first from the bone and then from the muscles, and to compare the two experiences of movement.

The Bones of the Foreleg (Figure 4.5)

Tibia

The tibia is the straightest bone in the body, yet it is also a good example of the spiraling nature of bone. If you run your hand down a skeletal model, you will feel the slight spirals in the topography of the bone. The tibia carries approximately 90 percent of the weight of the body through the foreleg and is primary in stability. The bone consists of a straight shaft and an articular surface at each end. Observe the following important landmarks of the tibia:

- The inferior articular surface, the smooth concave surface at the bottom end of the tibia that receives the convexity of the talus.

- The anterior margin, a sharp ridge on the front of the shin.

- The medial and lateral surfaces, on either side of the anterior margin.

- The medial malleolus, the inside anklebone. It protrudes from the tibia, continuous with the inferior medial surface, and helps to form the tibiotalar joint with its articular surface.

- The tibial tuberosity, the wide and rough protrusion of bone just below the kneecap.

- The medial and lateral condyles, the widening plateaus on each side of the proximal end of the bone. They support the superior articular facet, which is the articular surface on the tibia for the femur. The facet is divided into two distinct surfaces, one medial (the larger of the two) and one lateral, by a small ridge called the intercondylar eminence.

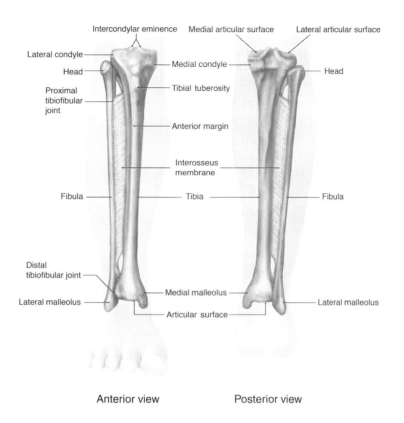

Intercondylar eminence   Medial articular surface   Lateral articular surface

Lateral condyle
Head
Proximal tibiofibular joint
Medial condyle
Tibial tuberosity
Head
Anterior margin
Interosseus membrane
Fibula
Tibia
Fibula
Distal tibiofibular joint
Lateral malleolus
Medial malleolus
Articular surface
Lateral malleolus

Anterior view   Posterior view

Figure 4.5

Tibia and fibula

Awakening the Tibia

Being large and available to touch, the tibia is a great bone for practicing skeletal touch and vibration with a partner. Referring to the practices outlined in Chapter Three, experiment with the following to help your partner embody the tibia:

- Mapping the tibia
- Cellular touch
- Vibrating the bone with your voice
- Touching the three layers of bone.

Fibula

Lateral to the tibia, the fibula also consists of a shaft with articular surfaces at both ends. However, the fibula is thinner and spirals more than the tibia: it carries only about 10 percent of the weight flowing through the foreleg, and is more related to fine-tuning of movement than to carrying the load. Identify the following landmarks on the fibula:

- Lateral malleolus: the distal end of the fibula, which serves as the lateral anklebone. With the medial malleolus of the tibia, the lateral malleolus forms a clasp or mortise within which the articular surface of the talus is able to glide.

- Head of the fibula: a protuberance lateral and slightly posterior to the tibia, just below the knee. It should have some freedom of movement when the knee is flexed.

Lying laterally and slightly posterior to the tibia just under the knee, the head of the fibula nestles into the tibia, beneath the lateral tibial condyle. When weight is not well centered in the leg, the head of the fibula can lose its mobility due to stresses on the ligamentous and muscular attachments. Working on releasing it can be very helpful in regaining full rotation in the foreleg.

Releasing the Head of the Fibula

On a partner's deeply flexed knee, locate the protuberance of the head of the fibula. Beginning with gentle touch, encourage the bone to move in relation to the tibia. Increase pressure as needed, and try approaching the movement through different layers of bone. Does moving the head of the fibula affect your partner's ankle?

Floating the Fibula

Positioning your partner in supine with a support beneath the knee, gently grasp the head of the fibula and with your other hand touch the lateral malleolus.

Connect the ends of the bone to each other with an energetic touch. Can you perceive the flow of energy through the bone? Then connect the ends of the bone to each other with a fluid touch. Can you perceive the flow of marrow through the bone?

Gently hold the bone at its ends as though it is floating free in space. Where does it want to go? Does it want to shift toward the heel, toward the pelvis, in rotation, or a combination of those movements? Follow the movement you perceive.

What is your experience? What is your partner's experience?

Mobility of the Foreleg

The tibia and fibula are a study in contrasts. The tibia is a strong, thick pillar for bearing weight, and the fibula is a slight, spiraling bone that makes the small adjustments that are necessary for gait and to adapt to the irregular surface of the earth. The two bones need to move in relationship to each other in order to sustain alignment, power, and flexibility in the lower extremities.

The tibia and fibula share distal and proximal articulations and are joined together by ligaments at each joint and by strong interosseous membranes between the bones. Despite the strength of those attachments and of the muscles that surround the foreleg, each bone has the freedom to rotate slightly around its longitudinal axis. The coordination of the longitudinal rotary movements in each bone creates mobility within the foreleg. When that movement is absent, or when one or both bones are locked in external or internal rotation, the holding in the bones of the foreleg contributes to the pattern of either supination or pronation in the foot (Figure 4.6). The same habit can contribute to discomfort at the knee and hip. While there are many possible patterns of rotation, you may be able to observe the following patterns in yourself and others.

- If the fibula rotates laterally (outward), the foot will respond with supination, the rolling under of the stable foot.

- If the fibula rotates medially (inward), the stable foot will be supported and the lateral foot will be stabilized.

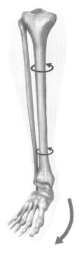

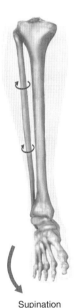

Pronation

Supination

Figure 4.6

Supination and pronation

- If the tibia rotates medially (toward midline of the body), the foot will respond with pronation, the rolling under of the mobile foot.

- If the tibia rotates laterally (toward the outside of the leg), the mobile foot will be supported and the medial foot will be stabilized.

Counter Rotation

When the motions of the tibia and fibula are balanced, they counter rotate efficiently during flexion and extension of the ankle. The motion provides equanimity in the joint space of the ankle and increases both range of motion and stability.

The motion of plantar flexion at the ankle is best supported by the outward counter rotation of the tibia and fibula—the tibia rotating medially and the fibula rotating laterally (Figure 4.7). That tiny motion has the effect of opening the front of the ankle joint and allows the front of the talus to glide forward freely, stay centered in the joint, and relate to the first three toes.

Similarly, the motion of dorsiflexion is best supported by the inward counter rotation of the

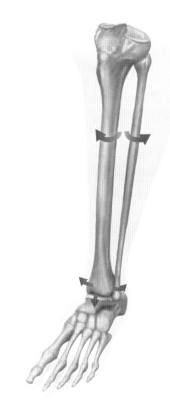

Figure 4.7

Foreleg counter rotation to support plantar flexion

bones toward each other—the tibia rotating later-ally toward the front of the ankle, and the fibula rotating medially (Figure 4.8). That tiny motion has the effect of opening the back of the joint, allowing the back of the talus to glide backward freely, and making the talus part of the heel with the calcaneus.

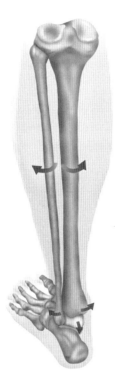

Figure 4.8

Foreleg counter rotation to support dorsiflexion

Foreleg Counter Rotation

Distal Movement at the Ankle

Sit comfortably so that you can support the bones of one leg with your hands. Initiate dorsiflexion at the ankle by imagining that

the tibia and fibula rotate toward each other to the front of the joint: support that motion with your hands. Let your talus follow the initiation by gliding backward in the joint, so that its articular surface peeks out toward the back.

In the same way, initiate plantar flexion by supporting the outward counter rotation of the tibia and fibula, closing the space at the back of the ankle and opening space in the front. Let your talus glide forward in the joint, so that its articular surface peeks out toward the front.

Proximal Movement at the Ankle

Stand in a comfortable parallel position of your feet. To produce dorsiflexion, a folding of the joint, initiate with forward counter rotation of the malleoli of your tibia and fibula. Again, you can feel that as a result of the excursion of the tibia over the talus, the posterior articular surface of the talus peeks out the back.

To return to standing from the folded position, initiate a backward counter rotation of the two bones. From standing, you can move into plantar flexion, rising on the toes to lift the heel off the floor, by continuing the balanced outward counter rotation of the malleoli of your tibia and fibula. Use the awareness of the two bones to control supination (falling onto the little toe side of the foot) and pronation (medial malleoli falling in toward each other) when your heel moves away from the floor.

Walking

After this exploration, take a walk, enjoying the mobility of your foreleg bones. Does movement in your legs feel free or constricted? Do your legs function symmetrically? Are the rhythms of movement the same?

Embodying the Knee

The knee is the largest and one of the most complex joints of the body (Figure 4.9). It addresses the demands of extreme mobility and stability, functioning equally well while bearing weight and moving freely in space. If the leg is a passageway between the trunk and the foot, the knee is the focal point of that passageway, as it permits multiple functions under tremendous stresses of weight and motion. In addition to providing the mobility associated with locomotion, the knee is adapted to work in conjunction with the ankle and hip joints to provide stability in standing. The movement of the knee produces a functional lengthening and shortening of the leg, modulating our relationship with the earth and our ability to move upon it.

The joint capsule contains two separate joints: the tibiofemoral and the patellofemoral, which together produce motions of flexion/extension and rotation. If you consider that the tibiofemoral joint is subdivided into medial and lateral

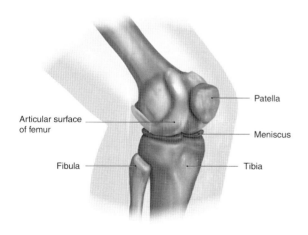

Fibula —

Articular surface of femur —

— Patella

— Meniscus

— Tibia

Figure 4.9

The knee

articulations, the knee actually has three joints. The bones of the knee form an inherently unstable joint, which is greatly strengthened by a robust joint capsule, many ligaments, and muscles working in harmony to surround and support the joint. Embodiment of the skeletal knee permits us to utilize it fully in both mobility and stability, and to mitigate the most extreme of the stresses that act upon it.

Bones of the Knee

Tibia

See *Bones of the Foreleg*, page 54

Femur

The femur transmits the weight of the body from the pelvis to the platform of the tibia (Figure 4.10). The largest bone in the body, it has a complex shape, bending through all three planes. Seen from the side, it is bowed to the front in the sagittal plane, like a bow with the hamstrings as the bowstring. Seen from the front, it has a sharp curvature in the vertical plane from its head to the medial epicondyle at its base, the primary weight-bearing surface. Seen from above, the epicondyles at the base of the femur are medially rotated in the horizontal plane, in relation to the neck and head. Landmarks to notice on the femur include:

The head

The rounded surface that articulates with the acetabulum of the pelvis.

The neck

A short protuberance that carries the head at an angle from the main shaft of the bone.

The greater trochanter

The large protuberance opposite the neck that is the site for many muscle attachments.

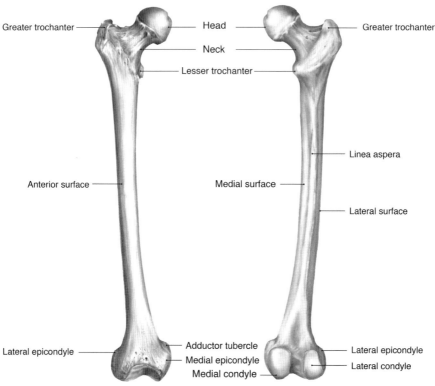

Figure 4.10

The femur

The lesser trochanter

A smaller protuberance on the medial surface of the shaft just underneath the neck. It is the attachment for the iliopsoas complex, the major flexors of the hip joint.

Three distinct shaft surfaces

Anterior, lateral, and medial.

The linea aspera

A ridge separating the lateral and medial shaft surfaces on the dorsal surface of the femur.

The medial and lateral condyles

The rounded articular surfaces at the distal end of the femur. The medial condyle is slightly larger than

the lateral. A space separates them posteriorly (inter-condylar fossa), and they are joined at the anterior or patellar surface. The condyles articulate with the superior articular facet of the tibia.

The medial and lateral epicondyles

Located at the distal end of the bone, they are not articular, but provide surfaces for attachment of muscles and ligaments. The medial epicondyle protrudes medially above the medial condyle. The lateral epicondyle rises above the lateral condyle, and is palpable as the first available bony surface on the distal and lateral thigh.

The adductor tubercle

A protuberance just above the medial epicondyle to which the adductor muscles attach. It is easily palpable on the medial and distal side of the leg, just above the knee joint.

Patella

The patella is a pebble-like bone embedded in the anterior knee joint. It serves as a pulley, increasing the angle and force directed onto the tibia by the quadriceps femoris ("quads") and reduces friction between the quadriceps tendon and the femoral condyles. Reflecting those two functions, the anterior surface is roughened, enabling ligaments and tendons to attach, and the posterior surface is smooth, allowing it to glide efficiently. In full knee extension, the patella sits on the anterior surface of the distal femur. With flexion, it glides down the femoral condyles. It has ligamentous attachments to the tibia that pull the patella across the distal femur. The patella rotates both medially and laterally.

Menisci

The menisci are half-moon shaped discs on the flat articular facets of the tibia that help to create sockets for the femoral condyles and provide cushioning, direction, and lubrication for movement. They are composed of cartilaginous connective tissue with a large amount of collagen fiber.

The medial meniscus is semicircular, wider at the posterior surface than at the anterior surface. It has widely separated attachments at the anterior and posterior surfaces, and also has an attachment at the medial collateral ligament. Because of those attachments, it is less mobile than the lateral meniscus. The lateral meniscus is more circular than the medial, with attachments that lie close together. Its width is consistent front to back. Because it is not fused with the lateral collateral ligament, it has more movement than the medial meniscus (Figure 4.11).

Front of knee

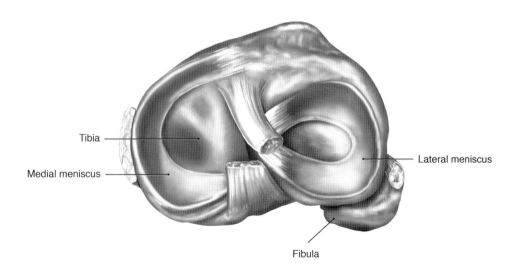

Tibia

Medial meniscus

Lateral meniscus

Fibula

Back of knee

Figure 4.11

Menisci of the right knee

Touching the Menisci

Invite your partner to sit in a chair with lower legs perpendicular to the thighs. With the fingers of both hands, find the tibial tuberosity below one knee. Carefully move your fingers toward the top of the tibia, where the hard bone stops and soft tissue begins, between the tibia and the kneecap. Gently press your fingers into that space, deeply enough to meet a resilient tissue that seems to bounce back when you release your touch. That is likely to be the anterior surface of the meniscus. Notice whether the two sides are similar or different: is one more present than the other and do they have the same degree of resilience?

Ask your partner what sensations emerge when you invite awareness into the menisci.

Movement of the Knee in the Planes

The dual articular surfaces of each knee move in extension/flexion through the sagittal plane, with the lateral and medial articular surfaces of each bone gliding over the corresponding surfaces of the other bone.

When the joint is in flexion, it can also move in internal/external rotation through the horizontal plane. During rotation, the lateral joint between the tibia and femur moves in the opposite direction from the medial joint. The joint is typically more limited by its ligaments in medial rotation than in lateral rotation. In full extension, the architecture of the joint does not allow for rotation.

Movement in the vertical plane (adduction/abduction) is severely limited by ligaments. Extreme pressure on the joint from either side causes a ligamentous injury.

The Knee in the Planes

Explore the range of movement in your knees in flexion/extension and rotation. Work with both distal movement and proximal movement. Enjoy their weight-bearing function and mobility. What do you observe about your knees? How do they feel? What are their habits?

Observing Movement in the Planes

Have your partner sit on a massage table or another surface where the foreleg and foot can dangle without touching the ground. Observe: notice how your partner arranges their body. Are the legs in abduction or adduction? Is the femur internally or externally rotating at the hip joint? Is the tibia internally or externally rotating at the knee?

Bring your partner's knees into line with the hip joint and the ankles, and observe the changes, the places of resistance, and what the felt sense of the joint is in the new position.

Gently move the lower leg in flexion and extension. Is the movement centered in the knee joint? Does the joint move freely in both directions, or is there a sense of constriction or resistance? How can you support the experience of equanimity of the joint with your hands?

With your partner's knee in flexion, gently move the tibia in external and internal rotation against the femur. Is there movement in both directions? Does the tibia seem to be already in rotation in one direction or the other?

What comes up for your partner in this exploration? Are any memories, sensations, stories, discomfort, or relief reported? What comes up for you?

The Role of the Menisci in Movement (Figure 4.12)

The flat plateau of the tibia alone does not provide a good receptacle for the rounded surfaces of the femoral condyles. Its slight concavity is improved and deepened by the semicircular menisci, which build up the edge of the tibial surface and help to form a limited socket for the balls of the condyles. If you make two O shapes with your index fingers and thumbs and hold the ends of the fingers together, you are approximating the shape of the two menisci. The femoral condyles would then sit comfortably in the deep receptacles made by your fingers and thumbs (Hartley, 1995, p. 143).

The attachments of the menisci to the tibia are approximately where your fingers and thumbs touch as you make the O. The ring of each meniscus is free to glide on the surface of the tibia. That freedom provides movement between the meniscus and the tibia as well as between the meniscus and the femur. The meniscus is free to move either with the tibia or the femur, and depending on the movement, the meniscus will join with either bone. In the movement of rotation at the knee, the menisci stabilize on the femur to glide as a single unit on the tibia. In flexion and extension, the menisci stabilize on the tibia to move as a unit around the femur.

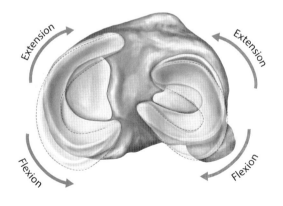

Figure 4.12

Movement of the menisci

During knee flexion, the bodies of the menisci rotate posteriorly on the tibia, while their attachments remain in place.

During knee extension, they rotate anteriorly on the tibia, while their attachments remain in place.

Initiation of Flexion and Extension from the Menisci

Sit on a table with your lower legs dangling over the edge. Slightly extend your legs, initiating from the anterior rotation of the menisci. Now lower your legs, initiating flexion from the posterior rotation of the menisci.

Walk, focusing on the flexion/extension of one knee, and feel the menisci initiating each movement.

How do those movements feel? What changes occur in your leg and the rest of your body as a result of initiating movement from the menisci?

Weight Flow Through the Knee

At the center of each knee is the intercondylar space, the gap between the condyles. When the weight-bearing line of force falls through that space, the result is a well-aligned and straight leg. When standing, sense the line of force falling through that space, as though you are standing on air. The chair and bubble images below will help you experience that sensation. If the weight-bearing line of force is displaced laterally, it runs more through the lateral femoral condyle or even the head of the fibula, possibly resulting in genu valgum, or knock-knees. If the weight-bearing line of force is displaced medially, it runs through the medial femoral condyle, with the possible result of genu varum, or bowed legs. Both variations place stress on multiple structures within the leg, and contribute to the deterioration of the cartilage on the articular surfaces of the knee.

Equanimity in the Knee: the Chair Image

To explore how weight flows through the bones of your knee in standing, it is helpful to think of the knee as a chair with four legs. Each leg is embedded in a corner of the knee, so there are medial and lateral front legs and medial and lateral back legs of the chair. Do any of the legs bear more weight than the others? Do any of the legs feel as though they are not supporting the weight of your body?

Now use the chair image with a partner. Ask your partner to stand in front of you. Lightly touch the four corners of the knee, as though you are supporting the four chair legs. Ask your partner to assess whether the weight falls evenly through each leg of the chair, or whether it seems that there is excess weight or no weight on one or more of the chair legs? Invite your partner to move sensitively to a position that allows weight to flow evenly through all four legs of the chair within the knee.

How does that shift affect the joint? How does it affect other parts of your partner's body?

Equanimity in the Knee: the Bubble Image

Another image to support ease in the knee is that of a soap bubble located in the center of the knee joint. Touch your partner gently and three-dimensionally around the knee, inviting the image of a tiny soap bubble at the center of the knee. Then ask your partner to allow the bubble to expand three-dimensionally until it is congruent with the surface of the skin at the knee. What part of the bubble is strong, and what part is weak? Does gentle touch register the same in all parts of the knee? If not, what adjustments need to be made such that the surface of the bubble feels even, and touch feels roughly the same over the entire surface?

When those adjustments are made, how do they affect the joint? How do they affect other parts of the body?

Traveling and Rotation of the Knee

In distal movement, the tibia travels around the femoral condyles (Figure 4.13). In proximal movement, the femur rotates on the surface of the tibia (Figure 4.14).

In flexion of the knee from standing (proximal movement), the entire knee moves forward in space. However, if we look during this movement at the knee joint alone, not at the spatial trajectory of the whole leg, we see that the tibia is actually moving backward in relation to the femur. In knee extension from a bent position in standing (proximal movement), the tibia is gliding forward (traveling) under the femur as the knee joint moves back in space.

The normal extension of the knee joint is 180 degrees. During the last 10 degrees of extension, the tibia rotates laterally (about five degrees of rotation). That is because the lateral femoral condyle, having a shorter and smaller surface, reaches its home position before the medial femoral condyle does. The small amount of gliding remaining to the medial condyle once the lateral condyle is home takes place in the horizontal plane, due to the slight rotation in the condylar surface.

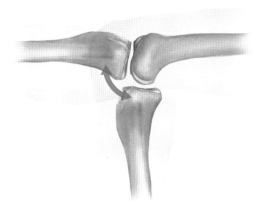

Figure 4.13

Traveling of the knee

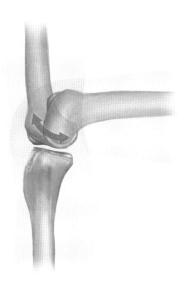

Figure 4.14

Rotation of the knee

Proximal Origination for Distal Movement: the Knee

Sitting in a chair, extend and release one leg at the knee. That is distal movement, since the femur is the support bone and the distal bone, the tibia, is moving. Now visualize the femoral condyles covered with velvet. Initiate the same movement from the feeling of the velvet surface, changing the direction of the nap in order to move the tibia. Does that change the quality of your movement?

Alternatively you might lie supine with your knees bent and one foot on the floor. Support the epicondyles of your lifted leg with your hands, aligning the hip, knee, and ankle joints. Imagine the rounded femoral condyles initiating the movement of your tibia, and visually track the movement of the foreleg as the tibia travels around the femur. Notice whether habits of rotation, abduction, or adduction limit the space within the joint cavity. How does it feel to enhance equanimity of the joint in traveling?

Distal Origination for Proximal Movement: the Knee

Kneel-sit on the floor. Rise from sitting on your heels to kneel-standing, and then come back down. That is proximal movement at the knee joint, since the tibia is the support bone and the proximal bone, the femur, is moving.

Now visualize the articular surface of the tibia covered with velvet. Originate the same movement from the feeling of the velvet surface, changing the direction of the nap. Does that shift in the initiation of the movement change its quality? Can you use that initiation to limit compensations such as the shoulders moving forward or buttocks moving backward? Your spine should be able to rise and descend without deviation from the vertical dimension.

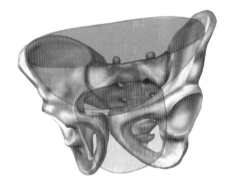

Figure 4.15

Two bowls of the pelvis

Embodying the Pelvis

The pelvic bowl is composed of four bones: the two pelvic halves (coxal bones), the sacrum, and the coccyx. Each coxal bone is formed from three separate growth plates, the ilium, the ischium, and the pubis, that do not fully harden into bone until about age 15 or 16. Our patterns of use therefore influence the shapes of our pelvic bones and joints. The female pelvis tends to be wider, adapted more towards stability and the demands of childbirth. The male pelvis tends to be narrower, adapted more towards mobility.

Mobility of the pelvis is dependent on movement at its joints: the right and left hip joints, the right and left sacroiliac joints, and the articulation of each pelvic half with the interpubic disc at the pubic symphysis. Some of us can even find wagging movement at the sacrococcygeal joint! The rotating counter movements of the hip joints, sacroiliac joints, pubic symphysis, and tail allow for the dynamic alternation of weight bearing and swinging of the legs, giving us the ability to walk on the earth.

When we examine the pelvis closely, we can see that there are actually two bowls in its structure (Figure 4.15). The iliac crests and the upper portion of the sacrum form a wide, shallow receptacle like a presentation bowl for fruit. A deep, narrow bowl is formed by the bottom of the sacrum, the ischium, and a part of the pubis—I think of this as a small mixing bowl.

Embodying the Two Bowls

Place your awareness in the upper part of your pelvis near your waist and the upper part of your pubic bone and sacrum. Visualize and feel the organs that reside there: the bladder, parts of the colon and small intestines, and uterus. Initiate movement from the upper bowl, the fruit bowl, allowing it to move forward and back, rotate, and tilt. Notice the sensations that it evokes and the responses in the rest of your body.

Then shift your awareness to the lower bowl, including the sitting bones, coccyx, ischium, and lower pubis. Within the small bowl are the rectum, anus, prostate, vagina, urethra, and muscles of the pelvic floor. Initiate movement from the lower bowl, allowing it to move forward and back, rotate, and tilt. How is this movement different from movement initiated from the upper bowl? How does your body react to each one?

Observed from above, the pelvis is divided into an anterior portion and a posterior portion. The anterior portion—which includes the pubis and ischial tuberosities—is more related to the function of the mobile foot. The posterior portion consisting of the ischial spine, ilium, and sacrum—is more adapted to the function of the stable foot.

Embodying Front and Back of Pelvis

In standing, emphasize the sensation of your stable foot: the two lateral rays with the calcaneus and cuboid. Enjoy the grounding this provides, and imagine lines of force that rise from the earth through your heel foot, lateral legs, and meet in your posterior pelvis, the sacrum. Widen your stance if you wish, bend your knees, and feel your stable-feet connecting into your posterior pelvis. What kind of action does this prepare you for?

Then bring awareness to your mobile foot. Begin walking, and imagine a flow from the big, second, and third toes upward toward the front of your pelvis—the pubis and ischium. Initiate forward motion from the front of your pelvis and see if the movement travels easily from there through your mobile foot.

Play with connecting your feet to your pelvis through the opposite patterns and see if they are more or less comfortable than the suggestions above!

Bones of the Pelvis

An individual coxal bone, or pelvic half, is a marvel of biological engineering (Figures 4.16, 4.17). It has three constituent bones, the pubis, the ilium, and the ischium, which are organized around the acetabulum, where they meet. The three bones fuse in childhood into the lightest structure possible through which tremendous forces can pass. The bone provides massive surfaces for muscle and ligament attachments, yet is delicate, with beautifully filigreed surfaces where the attachments are more minimal. Observe the thin and nearly translucent planar surface of the ilium, compared to the thickness of the weight-bearing passageway of the same bone between the acetabulum and the sacroiliac joint.

The edges of the pelvis form alternating concavities and convexities, as in the letter S, when seen from the proper angle.

Pubis

The pubis is shaped like a letter V placed on its side. The body of the pubis—the base of the letter V—is just lateral to midline of the body, forming a strong foundation that articulates with the opposite pubic bone at the pubic symphysis. The thick superior ramus emerges from the body as the horizontal portion that joins into the acetabulum. The more delicate inferior ramus descends from the body and reaches toward the ischium. Together the rami form two-thirds of the border of the obturator foramen, the hole just medial to the acetabulum.

Ischium

The ischium forms the base of the pelvis. It is composed of a body, a superior ramus, and an inferior ramus. The thick body forms part of the acetabulum: on its posterior surface, the ischial spine separates the greater sciatic notch from the lesser sciatic notch. The superior ramus projects downward from the body and includes a large swelling, the ischial tuberosity, or sitting bone. The inferior ramus of the ischium rises forward from the ischial tuberosity to meet the inferior pubic ramus.

Ilium

The ilium is divided into the body and the ala, or wing. The body forms part of the acetabulum, and is separated from the wing by a short, thick neck at the supra-acetabular sulcus. Locate the following landmarks:

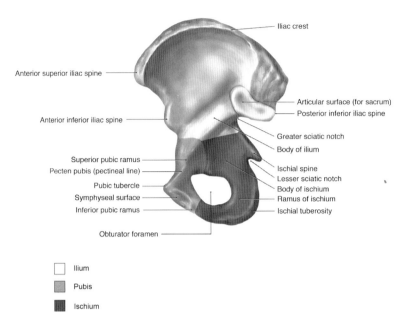

Figure 4.16

Coxal bone medial view

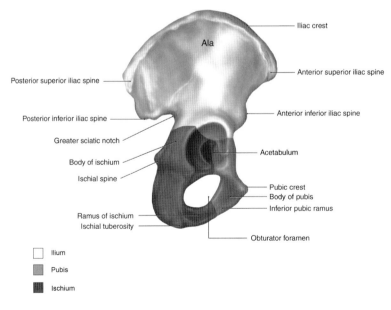

Figure 4.17

Coxal bone lateral view

The iliac crest

The top of the broad pelvic wing, surprisingly close to your waist and ribs.

The anterior superior iliac spine

An easily palpable eminence at the front of the iliac crest. Together the two anterior superior iliac spines are like headlights, shining forward through the darkness.

The anterior inferior iliac spine

Situated inferior and medial to the anterior inferior iliac spine, it is difficult to palpate, due to the musculature that lies over it.

The posterior superior iliac spine

An eminence at the posterior surface of the iliac wing. There is often a dimple at or just medial to the posterior superior iliac spine, which overlies the sacroiliac joint.

The posterior inferior iliac spine

An eminence that lies about one inch inferior and medial to the posterior superior iliac spine.

Sacrum

The sacrum, the sacred bone, is part of the axial skeleton (Figure 4.18). It also participates in the pelvic bowl. Like the talus in the foot, it is designed to shift easily between the functions of standing still and walking gait.

The sacrum is formed by the fusion of five sacral vertebrae. The bone is concave on its anterior surface. The wide base of the sacrum forms a support for the lumbar vertebrae. The narrower apex of the sacrum faces downward and articulates with the coccyx. When observed from above, one can see that the articular surface of the base is central and that large wings, the alae sacrales, emerge to the sides. They correspond to the transverse processes of the vertebral segments, but are greatly enlarged. Within the sacrum lies the sacral canal, an extension of the fluid-filled central canal of the spinal column. The four sacral foramina provide an exit for sacral nerves, both anteriorly and posteriorly. On the lateral aspect of the sacrum is a flattened auricular surface, so-called because it roughly resembles an ear. That rounded surface is covered with hyaline cartilage and forms a synovial joint with the neighboring ilium—the sacroiliac joint. Posterior to the auricular surface is the sacral tuberosity, a site for attachments for ligaments.

The triangular sacrum forms a wedge between the pelvic halves. That design transmits and distributes

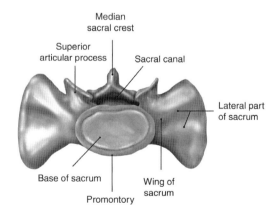
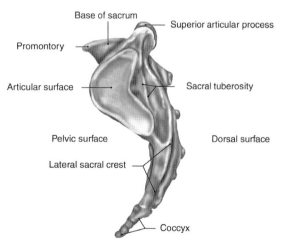

Figure 4.18

The sacrum

QR Code #5: Mapping the Pelvis

In walking or running the sacrum must constantly adjust its position to allow for the alternation of weight-flow into the legs. Its centrality both to contralateral movement and weight bearing makes it a key bone for human function. It is a truly sacred bone, as it facilitates the transcendent human traits of verticality and bipedal locomotion.

the weight of the spine and upper body into the pelvis and ultimately into the legs. In static weight bearing it is therefore the keystone of the weight-bearing arch of the pelvis (Dimon, 2011, p. 54). Its role is to transform skeletal forces from the single line of the axial spine into the dual force lines of the lower extremities.

To enhance the movement of the lower extremities it is vitally important to bring sensation, specificity, and awareness to the pelvis through sensory mapping. Bringing self-awareness to the pelvic bones involves touch around sensitive structures and should be done respectfully and gently, even with self-touch. Ensure that you do this work in a safe place, and take time.

Embodying the Pelvis: Bone Mapping

With a model or illustration of the pelvis available for reference, approach the pelvis from the navel, moving your fingers down to find the thick pubic crest or tubercle, above the pubic symphysis.

1. Lightly outline the contours of superior pubic ramus—both anterior and superior surfaces—as your fingers move toward the right ilium and back. Awaken the tissue of the periosteum with your touch. At a certain point near the acetabulum the bone will be difficult to map, as it is covered by muscle, ligament, and joint capsule.

2. Map the body of the right pubis, then walk your fingers down the ridge of the inferior pubic ramus. You may find it helpful to roll onto your left side and flex your right hip. Outlining the contour of the inferior ramus with your left hand, find the right ischial tuberosity (sitting bone) with your right hand. Map the bony bridge that connects your pubis with your sitting bone: your fingers will find continuity between the pubis and the ischial tuberosity of your right pelvic half. You are awakening the front of your pelvis.

3. With your right hand feel and enjoy the rounded surface of your ischial tuberosity. Then walk your fingers posteriorly and superiorly, up the posterior ischium. Depending upon the density of your musculature, you may be able to feel the lesser sciatic notch and the ischial spine. Eventually the bone dives underneath so much muscle that it becomes very difficult to palpate.

4. Shift your fingers to your right posterior inferior iliac spine, a protuberance just lateral to the sacrum. Find another prominence above that, the posterior superior iliac spine.

5. Map the continuity of the iliac wing as you move your fingers up and over the iliac crest, feeling its height and proximity to your ribs and waist. You may want to roll onto your back at this point.

6. Map the anterior superior iliac spine: it is the "headlight" of the pelvis, because it lights the way forward in space. Let your fingers feel the relationship between that landmark and the superior pubic ramus where you began the mapping.

7. Take some time to breathe into your bones. Initiate movement from your right pelvic half, enjoying the sensations of movement at the pubis, sacroiliac joint, and hip. Let the bone tissue tell you what it wants to do.

8. Stand and sense the difference between your right and left sides. How does it feel to walk? Has the mapping affected the fascial connectivity of your leg, your trunk, or your entire right side?

9. Repeat the mapping on the left side.

Neutral Pelvis

Alignment of the pelvis in standing or sitting refers to the even flow of weight through all parts of the structure (Figure 4.19). Deviations from the most efficient line of flow adversely affect pelvic joints and surrounding structures. In a functionally aligned pelvis—a neutral pelvis—the anterior superior iliac spines lie in the same vertical plane as the pubic symphysis. If the the anterior superior iliac spines and posterior superior iliac spines lie in the same horizontal plane the pelvis is in very slight retroversion: if the posterior superior iliac spine is very slightly higher than the anterior superior iliac spine the pelvis will be in neutral alignment.

Anterior and Posterior Pelvic Tilt

Anterior and posterior pelvic tilts occur when the relationship between the anterior and posterior iliac spines shifts out of neutral alignment. To sustain a tilt over time, compensation in the form of fascial, ligamentous or muscular strain is required in the hip joints, the lumbar spine, and the lumbosacral junction.

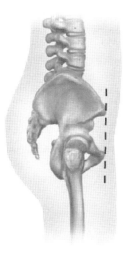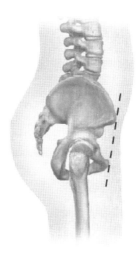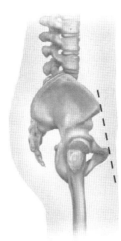

Figure 4.19

Alignment of the anterior superior iliac spine and pubic bone

In anterior pelvic tilt, also called anteversion, the anterior superior iliac spine moves in front of the pubic symphysis, which moves down while the posterior pelvis and posterior superior iliac spine rise. Relative to normal alignment, maintaining that position requires some degree of habitual flexion in the hip joint and an increase in the curvature of the lumbar spine (lordosis).

A posterior pelvic tilt (retroversion) moves the anterior superior iliac spine posterior to the pubic symphysis, which elevates while the sacrum and posterior supierior iliac spine depress. Maintaining that position involves an increase in extension in the hip joint and a decrease in the normal curve of the lumbar spine.

Anteversion and retroversion can be sustained on one or both legs and can be adopted as a foundation for movement in space. As a habitual stance, either one diminishes the normal movement of the pelvic bones, requires compensatory effort in walking and moving, and creates challenges to the alignment of neighboring joints.

Embodying Neutral Pelvis: Sitting

Sit with your ischial tuberosities toward the front of a hard, flat chair, avoiding use of the back support. Imagine the three curves of your spine floating up from the pelvis, like smoke rising from a chimney. Your shoulder joints are directly above your pelvis, not forward or back.

Feel the rounded surface of your sitting bones in contact with the chair. First ensure that you feel even pressure on each tuberosity—that may require some adjustment and relaxation in your organs and upper torso. Then roll your sitting bones forward as far as possible into extreme anteversion, maintaining your shoulders directly above your hip joints. Keeping your shoulders in the same position above your hip joints, roll back as much as you can on your sitting bones into retroversion, feeling how the position forces weight onto your gluteal muscles. Roll back and forth across the tuberosities in smaller and smaller increments until you find the center point between the two extremes. Check with your fingers to see if your two ASIS points and your pubic symphysis are in the same plane.

For many of us, this position of neutral pelvis in sitting will feel strange, more forward than usual. Others will feel a little more back. Breathe into the bowls of your pelvis and notice new sensations, adjustments, and responses in other parts of your body. If needed, take time for your muscles, fascia, and skeleton to unwind in this new spatial relationship.

Embodying Neutral Pelvis: Standing

Stand with your feet spreading into the earth and make sure that you are not locking your knees. Bring awareness to the alignment of your pelvis and the three curves of the spine floating above it, and let the front of your body release to the front while your back releases to the back.

Recall the points of contact on your sitting bones when you were sitting in neutral pelvic alignment: notice whether those same points on your sitting bones are directed back toward your heels or forward toward your toes. Allow those points to drop directly down over the center of your ankle joints. Notice what happens to your breath and flow of weight in your body when you do so. Once again check visually or with your fingers to ensure that your anterior superior iliac spine points are in the vertical plane with your pubic symphysis and that your posterior superior iliac spine are just slightly higher that the anterior superior iliac spine. How does that feel?

Lateral Pelvic Tilt

In a normally aligned pelvis, a line through the highest point on the iliac crests is parallel to the earth. Lateral pelvic tilt is a posture or movement in the vertical plane, where the two iliac crests are not horizontally aligned.

In a lateral tilt, one hip joint serves as the pivot point, and the iliac crest of the opposite side rises or drops around that pivot point. Elevating the opposite iliac crest creates abduction in the supporting hip joint, and the distance between the femur of the elevated side and the midline of the body is increased. Dropping the opposite iliac crest creates adduction in the supporting hip joint, and the distance between the femur and the midline of the body is decreased.

Lateral pelvic tilt may be related to uneven leg length or related to spinal abnormalities such as scoliosis.

Observation: Standing

Invite your partner to stand and to touch the top point of the right and left iliac crests. Are they at the same level? Is one higher than the other?

Identify the anterior superior iliac spine and posterior superior iliac spine of one pelvic half. Ask your partner to touch those points while you touch the same points on the other side, and observe.

Does one side appear rotated relative to the other? Is one pelvic half wider in front or narrower than the other is? Is one pelvic half wider in back or narrower than the other?

Observation: Folding

Invite your partner to bend forward as far as possible, first at the hip joint and then at waist. From the back, observe the symmetry or asymmetry of the pelvic halves in relationship to each other, while your partner is moving. Does one side initiate, elevate, rotate, or depress during the movement? Use touch at the iliac crests or posterior superior iliac spine to feel that process. If there is uneven motion can you and your partner identify the reason for its asymmetry?

Joints of the Pelvis

The Hip Joint

The concave receptacle of the acetabulum and the round head of the femur form the hip joint. The three bones of the pelvic half are not completely fused until the age of five to seven, and the acetabulum remains in development until the age of 15 to 16. The acetabulum lies at a downward and lateral angle, a perfect receptacle for the round head of the femur. Its bony wall is thicker on the superior surface (the roof of the socket). The concavity of the acetabulum is extended by the acetabular lip or labrum, a cartilaginous structure that is continuous with the acetabular surface.

The coxal bone appears as two planar surfaces, twisted counter to each other from their center at the acetabulum, organized like the rotary blades of an airplane with the acetabulum as the hub. The blades of an airplane engine provide forward thrust for the plane through space. Rotary movement of the coxal bone centered at the acetabulum does the same for us in locomotion.

When asked where their hip joint is, many people will point to the side of their pelvis, or to the greater trochanter. Establishing a clear sense of where the hip lies in your body is key to embodying movement at the joint and through the entire leg.

Embodying the Hip Joint

While standing or lying supine, gently flex and extend one leg at the hip and feel with your hands where the skin folds. At the level of the fold, gently place one hand on the inside of the leg and one hand on the outside of the leg. Then find the midpoint between these two places. Deep to your touch at the midpoint between front and back lies the hip joint.

Feel the relationship between the midpoint of the hip, the midline of the thigh, and the middle of the knee (the intercondylar space).

Breathe into the hip joint. Once again with your hand on the skin above the hip joint, flex and extend your hip, breathing into the sensation of movement within the joint. Can you feel the joint rotating deep to your fingers?

Compression and Release at the Hip Joint

Support the knees of a supine partner in anatomical position with a small bolster or towel. Identify both the greater trochanter and the site of the hip joint deep to the anterior surface of the joint: invite your partner to maintain self touch above the joint. Clarify for yourself the medial and superior direction from the trochanter through the neck into the head of the femur and acetabulum. Touching the trochanter, direct gentle pressure into the acetabulum until your partner is able to feel the head of the femur meeting the surface of the acetabulum. (I call it kissing!) Release the pressure and repeat several times, being careful not to press so hard that the compression travels into the sacroiliac joint. Check with your partner to ensure that they are feeling the location of the joint. When finished, invite your partner to move. See if your partner experiences any new awareness in the joint after the compression.

Movement of the Hip Joint

The hip joint moves in three degrees of freedom, with internal and external rotation, abduction and adduction, and flexion and extension. Those movements together permit circumduction, the movement in which the leg describes the surface of a cone, the apex of which lies in the head of the femur. From anatomical position, there is considerable flexion at the joint, but extremely limited extension. In distal movement, the femoral head rotates within the acetabular socket. In proximal movement, the acetabulum excursions around the femoral head.

Because of the oblique angle of the acetabulum, the entire femoral head does not articulate with the acetabulum in anatomical position. The greatest congruence between the head of the femur and the acetabulum occurs when the joint is internally rotated, slightly flexed, and slightly abducted. A familiar martial arts stance, that position provides the greatest stability in the hip joint.

When the center of weight bearing falls through the center of the femoral head, the joint can work with even and consistent motion. If the line of force falls either medially or laterally to that line, the joint will be compressed or limited in movement, as surrounding muscles are forced to tighten and compensate for the deviation. When the femoral head favors an anterior position within the hip joint, there will be limited external rotation in the joint, resulting in tight hips and the inability to let the hip joints fall toward the floor while seated.

Engaging Fluids in the Hip Joint

This exploration enhances synovial slipperiness within the joint. It feels great!

With your partner comfortably supine, position yourself carefully so that you can take the weight of the leg without straining your back. Support the leg with your shoulder, elbow, or hand under the knee, and encourage your partner to give you the full weight of the leg.

Slowly and gently move the leg through its range of motion. Allow your focus to be not on the leg, but on the space within the hip joint. Use small movement at first so that your partner's body can trust your rhythm, and gradually increase the speed and range of movement as your partner's body will allow.

Seek out the quality of sliding and gliding within the hip joint. Feel synovial fluid filling the joint space and improvise a little dance within your partner's joint from that sensation. How does the sliding and gliding feel to your partner? What difference does it make in standing and moving?

Rotating and Traveling at the Hip Joint

Rotation

Lying supine, with feet on the floor and knees toward the sky, release your weight into your sacrum and both sides of the pelvis. Flexing at the hip, simply raise one knee toward your chest, and listen for the feedback in your body. Notice how your body responds.

Shift your approach. Repeat the movement but initiate it by bringing your awareness to the femoral head rotating within the socket of the joint. Does that change your experience?

Traveling

Standing, release your weight into your feet. Bend forward as though you are going to touch the floor, and then return to upright position. Notice the sensations in your body as you move.

Shift your approach. Repeat the movement but initiate it by bringing your awareness to the traveling of the acetabulum over the femoral head. Invite the joint to fold deeply as the awareness of the gliding acetabulum increases. Use a similar deep initiation to rise back to standing. How does that change your experience?

Once you have felt the location of the hip joint and are clear about its rotation and traveling, you can further increase the equanimity within the joint by bringing greater specificity to the quality of initiation. At the hip joint, the distal bone is the femur and the coxal bone is proximal. If you originate movement clearly from the support bone, whether proximal or distal, the moving bone will glide more freely through its range of motion.

Distal and Proximal Originations for Movement at the Hip

Proximal Origination for Distal Movement

Lying supine, with your feet on the floor and knees toward the sky, feel into the depth of the acetabulum. Imagine that concave surface covered with velvet. Before moving the leg, imagine that the nap of the velvet will shift in the direction of the intended movement. When that image is strong in your felt sense, allow the femoral head to respond within the socket by rotating. How does that change your experience of moving your leg at the hip?

Distal Origination for Proximal Movement

Standing, feel the femoral head nesting deeply within the acetabulum, and sense its rounded form. Imagine the femoral head covered with velvet. Before bending the body forward by flexing the hip joint, imagine

that the nap of the velvet will shift in the direction of the intended movement. When that image is clear in your felt sense, allow the acetabulum to respond to the invitation of the velvet femoral head by traveling over it. How does that change your experience of moving your leg at the hip?

The Pubic Symphysis

The pubic symphysis forms the anterior joint between the two coxal bones. Its broad bony surfaces do not articulate with each other but with opposite surfaces of the interpubic disc that separates them. It is therefore actually two joints, with each side of the interpubic disc moving independently. Rotary motion at the joint occurs because of the counter motion of the coxal bones. Freedom at the pubic symphysis supports freedom of motion at the sacroiliac joints.

Embodying the Pubic Symphysis

Lie supine with feet on the floor and knees elevated. Place your fingers at your pubic symphysis, palpating the surfaces superior and anterior to the articulation. Alternately press your feet into the floor as though you are walking: with your fingers, feel the responses at the pubic articulations. Is the movement even? Do you feel more activity on one side of your pubic symphysis than on the other?

In table position, place one hand on your pubic symphysis. Alternately elevate and relax the knee on the same side as the supporting hand, ensuring that you have a nice lumbar curve to support the movement. Do you feel movement at your pubis with your fingers? Do the same on the other side: is there a similar sensation at the pubic joint, or is there a difference?

Finally, place your fingers on your pubic joints while walking. Notice the movement, lack of movement, symmetry, or asymmetry.

The Sacroiliac Joint

Movement at the sacroiliac joint is crucial for ease in walking and running. Although its range of motion is very small—two to 18 degrees of planar rotation—the joint's freedom sets the tone for movement through the whole leg. Traditionally considered a fused joint, it actually possesses synovial fluid and a joint capsule. Complete immobility is pathological, resulting from injury, lack of use, or other restrictions, and requires compensation in the musculoskeletal system at other joints. Some sacroiliac problems have to do with hyper-mobility, developed through extreme movement (either repetition or intensity) or through injury. In such cases, it is important to balance the forces around the SI joint and to support it muscularly.

Movement at the sacroiliac joint is closely associated with and affected by movement at the pubic symphysis and the hip joints.

Finding the Sacroiliac Joint

In standing, find the posterior superior iliac spine of both pelvic halves by placing your fingers on the dimple in the skin. Deep to those points are the centers of the sacroiliac joints. Shift your weight from foot to foot, and feel the response of the bones under your fingers.

Sacroiliac Range of Motion

It is helpful to feel the range of motion of the sacroiliac joint separate from the motion of the hip joint. Lying supine on the floor, center your pelvic weight evenly on the sacrum, and yield into the earth. Flexing at your hip, raise the extended right leg so that the foot is directed toward the ceiling. Center the foot directly over its hip joint, and renew the grounding of the sacrum into the earth. From that place:

1. Bring the right foot gently toward midline by adducting at the hip joint. Feel the limitation of the movement without releasing the right sacroiliac joint. Limit the motion to your hip.

2. Then allow yourself to widen to the right through your posterior pelvis and relax at the right sacroiliac joint so as to allow the foot to move further toward or across midline. Limit the motion to the right hip and SI joints.

3. Release at the left sacroiliac joint to further increase the range of motion of the leg. Allow the motion to include the hip and the right and left SI joints. You may even want to roll to the left as your leg goes further across your body.

What do you notice after this exploration?

Movement at the Sacroiliac Joints

Movement of the sacroiliac joint transforms somewhat from childhood into adolescence and adulthood. In children, the joint surfaces are smooth and permit gliding motions in all directions. With adolescence, the joint surfaces change to limit movement to counter rotation through the sagittal plane. The motion is called nutation and counternutation (Figure 4.20). In rare cases, if the supporting ligaments are lax or if great stresses suddenly impact on it, the adult sacroiliac can shear vertically, sliding

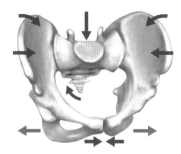

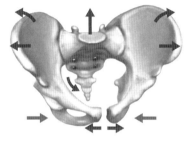

Figure 4.20

Nutation (above) and counternutation (below)

the pelvic half upward against the sacrum, or shear horizontally, sliding the pelvic half toward the midline of the sacrum.

In nutation at the sacroiliac joint, the apex (bottom) of the sacrum and the coccyx move posteriorly while the base (top) moves anteriorly. The distance between the coccyx and the pubis increases. (Visualize the tip of the tail moving backward away from the pubis.) Simultaneously the sitting bones move away from each other in the horizontal dimension, while the iliac crests at the top of the pelvis move inward, narrowing the waist. Together, those motions create a wider and deeper outlet at the bottom of the pelvis. An extreme version of that opening is achieved in childbirth. Nutation dilates the pelvic outlet, and supports flexion of the hip joints. If nutation is restricted as the leg moves into flexion, the movement will be governed by superficial muscles and less free as a result. When you embody the movement of nutation, the deeper musculature is engaged, liberating the more superficial

layers, and your leg will move easily through a wide range of motion (Franklin, 2003).

Counternutation is the opposite movement, in which the apex of the sacrum and the coccyx move anteriorly and the pubis moves posteriorly, so the distance between the coccyx and the pubis decreases. (Visualize the tip of the tail moving forward toward the pubis.) Simultaneously in the pelvic halves, the sitting bones move toward each other in the horizontal dimension, while the iliac crests at the top of the pelvis move outward, widening the waist. Together, those motions create a narrower and more constricted space at the pelvic outlet. Counternutation provides strength for the pelvic girdle, supports the stability of the standing leg, and is associated with hip extension. If counternutation is restricted, superficial muscles will be forced to over-work when stability is needed.

These subtle movements at the sacroiliac joint are only possible when the articulations at the pubic symphysis are moving as well. Movement at either joint requires a complementary movement at the other.

Initiating Movement with Nutation and Couternutation

Standing

With legs open slightly wider than the hips and externally rotated, bend your legs at the hips, knees, and ankles, and then return to standing. In dance, that is called a plié in second position. Try the same movement slowly, this time initiating from the widening and narrowing of the ischial tuberosities. Widening the tuberosities magically induces the hips to fold, the knees to move outward, and the muscles of legs to support but not to grip. Narrowing the tuberosities is similar and relatively effortless: by drawing them together you can return to a standing position without tightening your quadriceps. Can you feel the effortless quality of the plié?

With legs parallel and feet pointed forward, fold forward at the hip joint as far as is comfortable for your body and then return to erect posture. Then perform the same movement, initiating by increasing the distance between the coccyx and the pubis. Nutation will assist you in folding forward efficiently. Initiate the return to standing by decreasing the spaces between your pubis and coccyx and between your sitting bones (counternutation). You might feel that coming back to standing is effortless. What changes in your body and mind as you fold forward and return to standing in this way?

Lying Supine

Begin with your feet elevated in extension, legs either free in space or supported by a wall. Widen the distance between your legs so that they move laterally into space (a dancer's second position), and then return to the starting position, noting which muscles and bones have supported the movement. Repeat the movement, but initiate the opening by widening the distance between the ischial tuberosities, and initiate the return by narrowing that distance. How does that change your experience? What other structures become more active or less active when you initiate movement from your sitting bones?

Reciprocal Motion of the Sacroiliac Joints

In contralateral gait, there is a need for stability in the standing leg and mobility in the swinging leg. As a result, the SI joint of the support leg needs to be moving into counternutation, increasing stability in extension, while the sacroiliac joint of the swinging leg needs to be moving into nutation to support the flexion at the hip. The process reverses as the legs change roles: the sacrum participates in nutation on one side and counternutation on the other. The alternation of those opposite sacroiliac rotations permits the pelvis to move forward in space over the supporting legs.

In yoga, dance, and athletics the embodied use of reciprocal sacroiliac motion helps to increase range of motion when in lunge positions and stabilizes the body when balancing on a single leg. While the applications of this are almost infinite, a couple of examples are suggested below as starting explorations.

Reciprocal Movement in Nutation and Counternutation

Yoga: Tree Pose (Vrksasana)

Ballet: *Passé* or *retiré*

When standing in any version of tree pose or *passé*, become aware of the direction of counternutation of the sacroiliac joint in the standing leg and nutation in the bent leg. It is sometime helpful to reduce this to the sensation of narrowing your standing sitting bone toward midline while releasing the sitting bone of your lifted leg away from midline. Does this change the stability, ease, or flexibility of the pose?

Yoga: Warrior Pose (Virabhadrasana)

Ballet: Fourth Position Lunge

In any version of lunge, one leg is elongated and the other is flexed at the hip and knee. The elongated leg is in extension at the hip joint, so it is the standing leg. The flexed leg is actually your working leg. While moving into the pose, invite the sitting bone of the standing (back) leg to narrow toward the midline while allowing the sitting bone of the bent leg to flow into nutation, widening toward the knee. You may find that this allows your pose to deepen without increasing strain on your joints.

Try applying this idea to other poses and movements with asymmetry in the legs.

Walking

Place your hands on the dimples of your skin that lie above your posterior superior iliac spines. As you walk, can you feel the reciprocal movement of the sacroiliac joints? You will feel muscles moving as well, but invite your fingers to observe the movement of the bones. Is the range of movement even on each side, or does one seem to be freer than the other? If it is uneven, what else can you observe about each leg and the joints below?

Observation of Walking

From the back, the front, and the sides, observe a partner walking. First note how it makes you feel in your own body. What qualities does it evoke? Does the sacroiliac joint allow the stride to be free? Does it allow the gait to be even in rhythm and in space? Is there fluidity through the joint, or is there constriction? What do you notice about the relationship of the sacroiliac to your partner's other joints?

Bone Breathing in the Sacrum

Position your partner on his side or supine. If supine, ask permission to insert your hand underneath the pelvis, either from the side or from the direction of his tail. Your partner can help you position your hand comfortably. When you are positioned in a way that is comfortable to both of you, invite your partner to allow the sacrum to fall into your hand. If your partner is side lying, ensure that both of you are in comfortable positions.

Bring your awareness first to your own cellular breathing and particularly to the breath in your bones. When your own breathing is well established, renew your awareness of your partner's sacrum, and settle into an awareness of the bone breathing in a subtle expanding and condensing rhythm. If the bone wishes to move, follow the movement. If it remains resting, enjoy the contact and notice what changes in each of you.

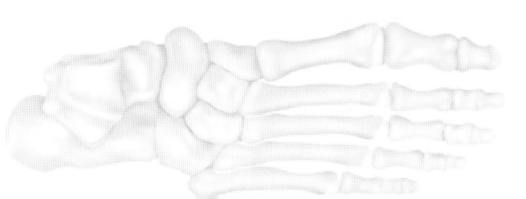

Decompression of the Sacroiliac Joint

Decompressing the sacroiliac joint can help to redirect the flow of weight through the pelvis and legs, and create space in the joint if there has been excess compression and lack of movement.

With your partner lying supine, place one hand under the sacrum, as described above. With your free hand, locate the iliac crest of the pelvis. With a very light touch (like a whisper), encourage the iliac crest to rise and rotate toward your partner's midline. You are not pushing! Your focus can be on creating space in the joint that is in contact with your supporting hand. Take your time, and work very gently.

Invite your partner to notice whether there are any changes in the experience or sensation of the joint.

Levering from Hip to Sacroiliac

With a supine partner, identify both the greater trochanter and the site of the hip joint with the leg in anatomical position. Clarify in your mind the medial and superior direction from the trochanter through the neck of the femur into the head of the femur. Compress slowly and gently in that direction until your partner is able to feel the head of the femur pressing into the acetabulum. Sensitively continue the compression. Follow the force of the pressure through the bone until you sense that the ilium has pressed gently into the sacrum at the SI joint. Allow a gentle release and expansion in the same slow rhythm. How does that feel, both for you and for your partner?

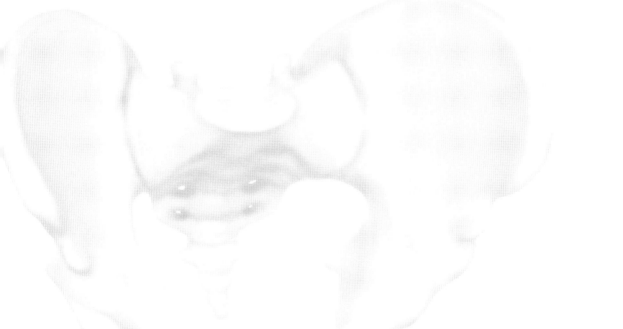

Integration: Foot to Pelvis

Bringing awareness to a single joint can create a ripple effect of consciousness through the body like a pebble dropped into a still pond, yet we cannot easily invite systemic change if the focus remains on single joints or bones. Having individuated the bones, we now want to integrate the lower extremities as a system. We will consider general principles of alignment, integration of the mobile foot and stable foot with specific parts of the coxal bone, and specific lines of connection from individual toes to the coxal bone.

Alignment of the Lower Extremities

The idea of a neutral, functional alignment is based on the architectural and structural potentials—the divine architecture—of the human body. No living human displays a completely neutral stance and gait. One of my first somatic movement teachers showed me an image of a human with ideal skeletal alignment. When I said that I'd like to be that way, she said that with an ideal form like that there would be no need to spend time on the earth: that person would just take a breath and go straight to heaven! I understand her point. Working toward ideal alignment is merely a construct that helps us organize as efficiently as possible given the constraints of age, bone growth, our responses to the environment, and the tone of our own nervous systems. Variation from the neutral is actually what makes us beautiful, what brings individuality and differentiation.

The human experience is that our responses to injuries, stressors, gravity, repetitive movement, and other influences gradually force us to deviate from the neutral. Over time, the body creatively constructs patterns of compensation in posture and movement, involving excess or deficient tone in the softer connective tissues around the bones and in growth and wear patterns of the bones themselves. Repatterning movement is not simply physical. It invites us to acknowledge what is being held in the tissues emotionally and psychologically. This is important in the lower extremities: they are the basis of your body's relationship to the earth, the way you walk in the world, and how you move toward and away from others.

Neutral Alignment

As mentioned briefly in Chapter Four, neutral skeletal alignment is based on anatomical position. The feet are in parallel directly beneath the hip joint with knees and toes directed forward. In that stance a plumb line falls from the articulation at the hip through the ray of the second toe, passing through the intercondylar space at the center of the knee and the center point of the ankle (Figure 5.1). When weight flows through those points, the ischial tuberosity rides directly over the medial epicondyle of the femur and the medial malleolus of the tibia. Variations from that optimal plumb line are infinite, but may include the following:

- Internal or external rotation of the femur at the hip
- Internal or external rotation of the tibia and/or fibula in relationship to the femur
- Adduction or abduction of the femur at the hip and/or the tibia at the knee resulting in genu valgus or genu varus
- Hyper- or hypo-extension of the knee
- Pronation or eversion of the foot
- Rotation, narrowing, or widening of the pelvis at either or both sacroiliac joints.

A variation at any level or joint necessitates compensation in neighboring joints as well as in the fascial web and supporting ligaments. Therefore, a pronated foot is not just a pronated foot; it is part of a system that includes the ankle, foreleg, knee, and hip, if not more of the body. We can encourage optimal function and the pronated foot toward a more neutral alignment by directing attention to each part of the whole.

Many of us identify such variations as states of being: "I'm flat-footed" or "I'm bow-legged." It might be more helpful to see those traits as habits of movement and alignment, or deeply rooted choices within ourselves. That perspective creates the possibility of changing movement or postural habits slowly over time, and changing the very structure of the bones. Bones are continually reforming themselves at a cellular level in an ongoing dance of death and rebirth. They respond to the stresses placed on them by the forces of the earth, our muscles, and our activities by reinforcing the density of bone where it is needed and reshaping themselves toward patterns of use. To the degree that mindful movement is habitual, you invite your bones and their accompanying fascial web to reshape themselves and move toward a more neutral alignment. Change happens!

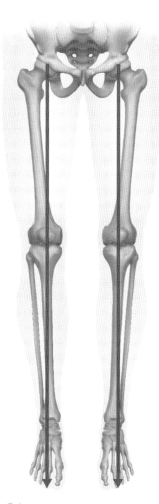

Figure 5.1

Plumb lines

Standing with a Mirror

Stand in parallel position in front of a full-length mirror. To the best of your abilities, establish clear plumb lines through the center of your hip joint, knees, and ankles. Notice the sensations associated with that stance and how they may be different from your habitual stance.

As you observe yourself, what do you see? Are your feet and lower legs internally or externally rotated, or are they parallel? Are your feet pronated, supinated, or balanced?

If there is a tendency toward pronation or supination, how does that affect the plumb line through your knees? Are your pelvic halves symmetrical or asymmetrical?

What else do you notice in the descent of weight through your legs? Compared to your habitual stance does this feel more grounded or less, more vulnerable or less, more effortful or less?

Observation with a Partner

Because our bodies perceive our idiosyncrasies as normal, it can be helpful to discuss the questions posed above with a partner. Take care to give and receive the feedback non-judgmentally. You are simply acquiring information that can be useful for repatterning your movement.

Having established the feeling of a neutral alignment in standing, try walking. The plumb line also informs the relationships among the joints as you move in space. To sustain it, sagittal plane motion at each joint is essential: the hip, knee, and ankle are designed to fold and unfold in the sagittal plane. If your gait displays deviations from sagittal plane motion in those joints, however subtle, the movement requires greater muscular effort, strain through the fascial system, and lengthening and shortening of ligaments that would prefer to remain balanced.

Imagine that each of those joints is a wheel on a train. Forward motion requires the wheel to stay aligned on the railroad track. If it deviates, it will experience friction, wear down, or go off the track entirely. In your joints, those deviations eventually create pain, arthritis, and stiffness. Keep your joints on track!

Walking the Railroad Tracks

With a mirror or a partner, stand with your feet in neutral alignment beneath your hip joints. Imagine that your plumb lines continue forward along the floor as if they were parallel railroad tracks. (Sometimes the seams in wooden floors provide nice analogs to tracks.) Walk normally and observe your habits of alignment in movement. Do your hips and knees fold and unfold simply and elegantly? Do your forelegs swing outward from the knee, or remain in parallel alignment through the movement? Do your legs perform extra rotations at ankle, knee, or hip? Do your feet comfortably align themselves on the tracks, or do they prefer external or internal rotation?

Then walk and see if you can adjust your gait so that each joint moves forward along on the track without deviation. It may be difficult to balance: some people have the feeling that they are babies learning to walk all over again. Notice whether any adaptations to your normal gait would easy for you to practice. Your body will welcome the change.

Integration of Mobile Foot and Stable Foot to Pelvic Half

The anterior pelvis and the mobile foot are both adapted for mobility. The posterior pelvis and stable foot are inherently stable. We can look at the foot and pelvis not as distant body parts but as companions within two functional systems: the mobility system and the stability system, each one continuous from a foot to the pelvic half of the same side. Two pathways, one direct (Table 5.1) and one spiraling (Table 5.2), connect the mobile foot to the anterior pelvis and the stable foot to the posterior pelvis. Each one has different advantages and can be used for different purposes. The pathways begin and end at the same points; the differences are highlighted in the charts below (Bainbridge Cohen, 1995, pp. 5-6).

Table 5.1: Direct Pathways: Mobile Foot and Stable Foot to Pelvic Half

	Mobile Foot Pathway	Stable Foot Pathway
Foot	First three toes	Fourth and fifth toes
	Metatarsals	Fourth and fifth metatarsals
	Cuneiforms	Cuboid
	Navicular	Calcaneus
	Talus	
Foreleg	Tibia	Fibula
Knee	Medial femoral epicondyle	Lateral femoral condyle
	Inside pathway on femur and lesser trochanter	Iliotibial band and greater trochanter
Pathway ends	Superior pubic ramus on same side	Spiraling back to sacroiliac joint on same side

Table 5.2: Spiral Pathways: Mobile Foot and Stable Foot to Pelvic Half

	Mobile Foot Pathway	Stable Foot Pathway
Foot	First three toes and metatarsals	Fourth and fifth toes and metatarsals
	Cuneiforms	Cuboid
	Navicular	Calcaneus
	Talus	
Foreleg	Medial malleolus of tibia spiraling around the front to head of fibula	Lateral malleolus of fibula spiraling back around tibia to medial femoral condyles
Knee	Spiral around back of knee	
Femur	Spiraling from posterior to medial side of femur	Spiraling from medial femoral condyles around front of femur to greater trochanter
Pathway ends	Superior pubic ramus on same side	Spiraling from greater trochanter to sacroiliac joint on same side

Integration of Foot to Pelvic Half: Movement Practices

QR Code #6: Lower Extremity Alignment

Movement Exploration: Mobile Foot to Pubis in Prone Position

Lying on the floor in prone position with legs in parallel, tuck your toes under so that the underside of the big toe is in contact with the floor, emphasizing the alignment of your mobile foot. Initiate a gentle push from the toe. Where does the movement travel in your leg, and where in your pelvis or back does it arrive?

Initiate the movement again, and carefully track the pressure from your big toe moving into the cuneiforms and navicular, into the talus, through the medial side of the tibia and the medial femoral condyle, and finally into your pubis and pubic symphysis. Does this change the lines of force in your legs? How does it affect the rest of your body?

Movement Exploration: Foot to Pelvis Integration While Standing

Standing in parallel, center your feet underneath your pelvis. Press into your toes so that your heels lift off the ground (*relevé*, in dance). Be aware of the force of gravity rising from the earth through the mobile foot, connecting through the direct pathway of your medial bone structure to the anterior pelvis. Try both pathways, direct and spiraling, and see which works for you, or if you perceive an entirely different pathway.

From the same starting position, fold your ankle, knee, and hip so that your body releases toward the earth, yielding your weight through the bones. Invite weight to flow from your sacroiliac joint down to your heel foot, connecting the bony structure of stability through the lateral leg. Another option is to try the spiraling pathway, flowing from sacroiliac around your trochanter toward the medial knee, then spiraling around the posterior foreleg and into the ankle foot.

Walking Foot to Pelvis Integration

Walk normally. Sensing your foot, notice whether it utilizes both mobile foot and stable foot during your stride. Feel whether the pelvis is balanced between stability and mobility (back and front), or whether one function is favored over the other.

Integration of Foot to Pelvic Half: Hands-On Practices

Bone Mapping

With a partner, use your hand or a soft brush to map the bony pathways in one leg from toes of the mobile foot to the anterior pelvis and from toes of the stable foot to the posterior pelvis. Have your partner stand and compare the sensation of the mapped leg with that of the untreated leg before you trace the pathways in the other leg.

Levering Through the Bones

Position a small pillow or bolster under the knees of a supine partner. Placing your hands on the mobile foot, create a gentle compression into the ankle joint. Sustaining that pressure, guide the flow of compression into the medial knee, adjusting your hands as necessary to support that pathway. Then see if you can thread the compression through the medial thigh into the anterior pelvis and pubic symphysis. Release the pressure and allow the joints to expand. Assess whether it would help to reposition your partner to obtain a more efficient line of force from mobile foot to pubis.

In the same way, use gentle compression of the stable foot into the talus and then toward the fibula. Allow the sequence of compression to thread its way through the bones and tissues of the lateral leg into the posterior pelvis and sacroiliac joint.

Invite your partner to stand and walk, and to feel if there is a change in the felt sense of the leg as a result of differentiating the stability structure from the mobility structure.

Lines of Connection from Toes to Pelvic Half (Table 5.3)

We can refine the stability and mobility pathways by specifying the relationships between the individual toes and corresponding regions of the pelvis. Bonnie Bainbridge Cohen teaches that defining those relationships further clarifies foot–pelvis integration, both in standing and in locomotion. The chart below, based on her investigation, presents a set of relationships between individual toes and specific areas of the pelvis. Through your own experimentation, see if those relationships hold true for your body.

Table 5.3: Lines of Connection from Toes to Pelvic Half

Toe	Pelvic Half
Big toe	Superior pubic ramus and pubic symphysis
Second toe	Inferior pubic ramis to ischial tuberosity
Third toe	Center of acetabulum
Fourth toe	Posterior portion of ischial tuberosity to spine of ischium
Fifth toe	Posterior iliac crests and sacroiliac joint

Toes to Pelvic Half: Movement Practices

Standing Toes to Pelvic Half

Gently press your big toe into the floor, while touching the pubic crest of the same side. Move in place or walk, sensing the line of connection between those points.

Gently press the second toe into the floor, while touching or feeling the inferior pubic ramus and ischial tuberosity. Move again, sensing the connection through the leg between those points.

Gently press the third toe into the floor, while touching or feeling the skin above your acetabulum. Sustain the connection between those points as you walk and move.

Gently press the fourth toe into the floor, while touching the posterior part of your ischium. Shift from side to side, sensing the connection through the leg between those points.

Gently press the fifth toe into the floor, while touching or feeling the PSIS and your skin above the sacroiliac joint. Shift your weight and stand on the leg as you feel the connection between those points.

Symmetrical Limb Sequencing, Feet Against the Wall

Lie on your back with your feet against a wall, hips and knees at right angles and centered on your sacrum. In this resting position, check the plumb lines from your hips through second toes, relax your feet, and establish a relationship between your sitting bones and heels.

Maintain the relaxation of your feet as you press your toes into the wall to feel the lines of connection into the pelvis. Yield your feet even more deeply into the wall as you engage a whisper of a push, first in your ankles, then knees, and hips. When the increasing tone arrives in your pelvis slide away from the wall as your feet stay relaxed and connected with the wall. Track the evenness or asymmetry in your joints as you move. Try to initiate and follow through in a perfectly symmetrical movement. Notice if any joint wants to deviate from the plumb line, and remember the feeling of walking on the railroad tracks: this is similar, but in service of symmetrical movement instead of alternating gait.

Toes to Pelvic Half: Hands-on Practices

The following explorations are options for eliciting awareness of the lines of toe to pelvis connection in your partner's body. You may also do the touch explorations on yourself. The standing exploration transitions easily into further exploration through movement. The supine exploration allows the recipient of touch to be more fully sensory.

Touch Exploration: Toe to Pelvis Integration While Standing

Using your fingers or a brush, trace the line of connection between each toe and its related region on the pelvis. Experiment with finding pathways both in the front and the back of the leg and foot. Assess what the sensory change is in the receiving partner, and how the touch affects their stability and mobility. Compare sensation in the leg that has been touched with that in the leg that has not yet been touched.

Touch Exploration: Toe to Pelvis Integration While Lying Down

Have your partner lie supine. With a brush or your fingers lightly chart the line of connection between each toe and the related region of the pelvis, making sure to find a continuous pathway. Don't worry about the correct path; find a route that makes sense to you and your partner. Try charting a course on the back of the leg as well as the front. Adjust to your partner's appetite for touch: deeper, lighter, faster, slower. Adjust your partner's position on the floor to facilitate the changing pathways. Complete one leg and compare its sensation to that of the untreated leg. Invite your partner to stand and see what the effect is on the entire body before changing sides.

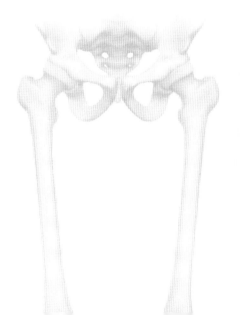

The Upper Extremities

Our upper extremities—hands, forearms, arms, shoulder girdle, sternum, and ribs—can push, pull, lift, hold, embrace, knead, grasp, release, snap, tap, clap, thread, throw, cut, strike, pinch, brush, and pour, to name some of the movements we perform on a daily basis. In many cultures and languages, the hands mirror or even precede the voice in speech, and in the case of sign language they are used as eloquently as the voice.

Unlike most other mammalian species, the upper extremities in humans are not used primarily for locomotion but for interacting with the environment. Most of our upper extremity bones and joints are better adapted to mobility than to bearing weight. While our feet and legs allow us to move upon the earth, our hands and arms allow us to act on the environment. Our hands can move seamlessly and omni-directionally in space—from near to far, from up to down, from midline to lateral, in pronation or supination—and they are able to perform an infinite variety of tasks, thanks to our uniquely human opposable thumb.

Embodying the Hand

The skeletal map of the hand recalls that of the foot in many respects, but with some important adaptations: the phalanges of the fingers are longer than those of the toes, the metacarpals of the hand are more delicate than the metatarsals of the foot, and the carpal bones at the wrist are smaller and function more as a unit than the tarsal bones of the foot.

Then there is the thumb. Unlike the great toe of the foot, the thumb of the hand has the ability to rotate and face the other digits, giving us the capacity for precision in grasping. The thumb is one aspect of our skeletal system that makes us unique in the animal kingdom: no other mammal has developed the dexterity that we possess as a result of our movable thumb.

As we begin to look at the skeleton, consider your own hands. What is their history? What activities of daily life do they perform well, and what is a challenge? Are you a knitter, a woodworker, a typist, a painter? What do your hands do every day: wash dishes, open doors, pick up a phone, prepare food, reach for a high shelf? Do they make music? How do you use them in relating to others? Do you use them as part of your expressive speech? Have they sustained breaks? Warts? Pain? What are the characteristics of your hands? Which hand is dominant? Do you hide them, or make judgments about their appearance?

If each hand had a voice, what would yours say to you?

Observing Hands

Observe the hands of many people, both at rest and in motion. What do they express? Are their bones long and thin, short and thick, or something in between? What is your general impression of the hands, and how they move? Do the subjects use them to emphasize or support speech, or is their movement limited? What is the personality of the hands, and what do they express about the person?

The Bones of the Hand (Figure 6.1)

Phalanges

The phalanges are the bones of the fingers. The thumb has two phalanges, distal and proximal. The remaining four fingers each have three: distal, middle, and proximal. Each phalanx has a proximal base, a shaft and a distal head. Joints between the phalanges are called interphalangeal joints, which move only in flexion and extension.

Metacarpals

The metacarpals are the five bones of the palm. Each finger has a metacarpal bone at its base, numbered from first—the thumb—to the fifth. Each metacarpal bone has a distal base, a shaft, and a proximal head. The joints between the phalanges and the metacarpals are the metacarpophalangeal joints, which move in flexion/extension and abduction/adduction. The heads of the metacarpals have joints with each other, with articular facets providing little movement. At their proximal ends the metacarpals are joined to the carpals by strong ligaments at the carpometacarpal joints. The thumb's carpometacarpal joint is saddle-shaped, allowing abduction and adduction as well as opposition and circumduction. The second and third carpometacarpal joints are essentially non-moving, providing stability for the hollow of the palm. The fourth has a small but appreciable range of motion in flexion and extension. The fifth carpometacarpal has a greater range of motion than the fourth, and is able to slightly abduct and adduct as well.

Carpals

The carpals are the eight bones of the wrist that together form a concave arch on the palmar surface (Figure 6.2). As a unit, they are called the carpus. Tightly packed, each bone has multiple facets for articulating with neighboring bones. These tiny, pebble-like bones sit in two rows of four bones each, a proximal and distal row, forming the midcarpal joint.

Carpal Bones, Proximal Row

Scaphoid

Named for its resemblance to a boat, the scaphoid is the most lateral and the largest bone of the proximal row, positioned at the base of the thumb, index, and middle fingers. The scaphoid articulates proximally at the wrist joint with the radius, distally with the trapezium and trapezoid, and medially with the lunate and capitate. On the palmar side is a tubercle that is easily palpable through the skin. It is the most frequently fractured of the carpal bones.

Lunate

Shaped like a crescent moon, the lunate is the second bone in the proximal row. Positioned at the base of the rays of the fourth and fifth fingers it

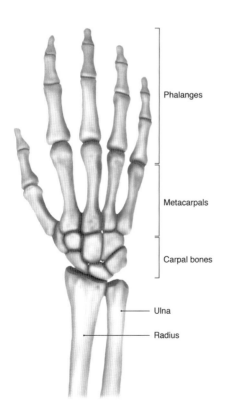

Phalanges

Metacarpals

Carpal bones

Ulna

Radius

Figure 6.1

Bones of the right hand, dorsal view

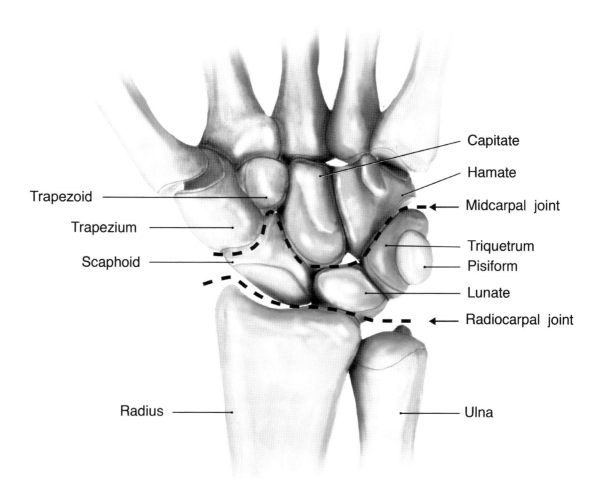

Figure 6.2

The carpal bones

articulates proximally with the radius and articular disc, medially with the triquetrum, laterally with the scaphoid, and distally with the capitate.

Triquetrum

The three-cornered triquetrum is the third bone in the proximal row. It is pyramidal in shape, with its apex directed medially. Its lateral surface articulates

with the lunate. It articulates proximally with the articular disc, distally with the hamate, and anteriorly with the pisiform.

Pisiform

Resembling a pea, the pisiform is the smallest carpal. It is rounded and articulates only with the triquetrum. In flexion it is easily palpable.

Carpal Bones, Distal Row

Trapezium

The trapezium is the most lateral bone in the distal row. It supports the thumb and transmits forces from the scaphoid into the first metacarpal and thumb. Distally, it forms a saddle-shaped surface for its articulation with the first metacarpal. Proximally, it articulates with the scaphoid. Medially, there is a facet for articulation with the trapezoid, and distal to that a small surface for a minor articulation with the second metacarpal.

Trapezoid

The second bone in the distal row, the small trapezoid is a quadrilateral bone having two parallel sides. It is wider on the dorsal surface and narrower on the palmar surface: its shape reinforces the arch of the carpus. It articulates proximally with the scaphoid, distally with the second metacarpal, laterally with the trapezium, and medially with the capitate.

Capitate

The capitate, the third bone of the distal row, is the largest of the carpal bones and sits in a central position in the carpus. It supports the third metacarpal, leading to the middle finger, and is key to balancing the forces through the hand: the capitate is the captain! It also articulates distally with the second and fourth metacarpals, proximally both with the scaphoid and the lunate, medially with the hamate, and laterally with the trapezoid.

Hamate

The hook-shaped hamate is the fourth bone in the distal sequence, and supports both the fourth and fifth metacarpals leading to the fourth and fifth fingers. It also articulates proximally with the lunate, and proximally and medially with the triquetrum. Its easily palpable curved hook, the hamulus, is on its palmar surface, serving as an attachment for the flexor retinaculum. (The flexor retinaculum is a ligamentous band that forms the carpal tunnel, stretching from the scaphoid and trapezium on the lateral side to the hamate, triquetrum, and pisiform on the medial side.)

Vibrating the Carpus

Enliven your carpal bones by using your voice to vibrate them. Placing your mouth on the bones, vibrate into every surface of the wrist, varying the intensity and pitch of your voice. Imagine that the sound is excavating the tiny spaces between the bones and then moving directly through the bones. Notice how your wrist feels before and after the vibration: it can be a helpful practice when taking a break from typing, writing, drawing, sewing, or any other activity that uses the hand intensively.

The Rays of the Hand

Just as the foot is organized into rays from the distal phalanges into the tarsal bones, the skeletal hand forms rays from its distal phalanges through the carpal bones. Each finger is the product of a sequence of bones traveling deep into the palm. The distal phalanges connect in sequence with the middle and proximal phalanges, into their respective metacarpals, and ultimately into the carpal bones to create radiating lines of energy from the wrist to the end of each finger.

Mapping the Hand

Using periosteal touch on yourself or a partner, map the bony ray of each finger from the distal phalanx to the head of the metacarpal and into the supporting carpal bones. Awakening the periosteum, map the contours of the carpal bones, individuating them. Find the capitate bone, and touch it with your fingers from above and below. You may be able to exert alternating pressure from each side and loosen the ligaments attaching it to its neighbors. Be sure to notice the effects of the mapping and get feedback from your partner about your touch and their experience.

Freeing Articulations Within the Hand

Sequencing through a partner's hand, gently move each joint through its full range of motion. Then compress and release the joint space. For the joints between the closely packed carpal bones, identify the joints and find where movement exists and where it is more restricted. In less mobile joints, you may want to work with cellular touch, to bring awareness. Be sure to get feedback from your partner about your touch and about their experience. How does the newly awakened hand feel compared to the unexplored one?

Radial Hand and Ulnar Hand

As in the foot, the hand uses two skeletal strategies to modulate between mobility and stability. The function of mobility is the province of the radial hand: the thumb side of the hand that emerges from the radial bone of the forearm. It is the radial hand that provides dexterity. Stability and strength are managed by the ulnar hand: the medial side that continues the line of the ulna in the forearm. In the foot, the delineation between the mobile foot and the stable foot is quite clear. In the hand, the middle finger and its supporting bones can shift to become allied with either the radial or ulnar hand,

depending on the movement and position of the wrist. The middle finger, third metacarpal, and capitate can also become independent of both skeletal structures to form a neutral axis of rotation for the wrist and forearm. The following are the components of the basic longitudinal groupings of the bones in the hand (Table 6.1, Table 6.2).

Prehension

Prehension is the use of the fingers and hand for taking hold of an object. The two major categories of prehension are the power grip, which emphasizes the use of the stronger ulnar hand, and precision handling, which emphasizes the use of the more articulate radial hand.

The Power Grip

The power grip utilizes flexion at all finger joints and often involves the palm. The power grip has a static phase, where the hand encloses an object, and force is maintained or increased. Flexion or deviation at the wrist diminishes the strength of the grip. There are three basic types of power grip:

1. Cylindrical grip, in which the thumb opposes the four fingers: the motion of gripping a baseball bat. The thumb can be in a variety of positions, but the phalanges of the fingers remain

Table 6.1: Bones of the Radial and Ulnar Hand

Radial Hand	Ulnar Hand
Phalanges of the thumb, index, and third fingers	Phalanges of the fourth and fifth fingers
First three metacarpals	Fourth and fifth metacarpals
Trapezium, trapezoid, capitate	Hamate
Scaphoid	Lunate, triquetrum, pisiform
	Articular disc

Table 6.2: Bones of the Radial and Ulnar Hand with Center Line

Radial Hand	Center Line	Ulnar Hand
Phalanges of the thumb and index fingers	Phalanges of the third finger	Phalanges of the fourth and fifth fingers
First two metacarpals	Third metacarpal	Fourth and fifth metacarpals
Trapezium and trapezoid	Capitate	Hamate
Scaphoid	Scaphoid and lunate	Lunate, triquetrum, pisiform
		Articular disc

parallel to each other. The stronger the grip, the more the hand will go into ulnar deviation, which is the most efficient position for the flexor muscles to act over the bone.

2. Spherical grip is similar to cylindrical grip, but the fingers are spread more and the hand surrounds a rounded object. This is the motion of holding a tennis ball.

3. Hook grip, which is primarily a grip of the fingers, as when holding an overhead strap in a subway car or a suitcase. It may include the palm but never the thumb.

Precision Handling

Precision handling is more variable than the power grip and requires much finer motor control and sensory awareness (Figure 6.3). In precision handling, the thumb forms one side of a pincer, like a pair of pliers, and is abducted from and rotated toward the palm. The other side of the pincer is formed by the tip, the pad, or the side of one or more fingers, leaving the palm free. There is generally more movement and less static contraction in precision handling than in the power grip. There are three basic types of precision handling, which in infancy develop in the following order:

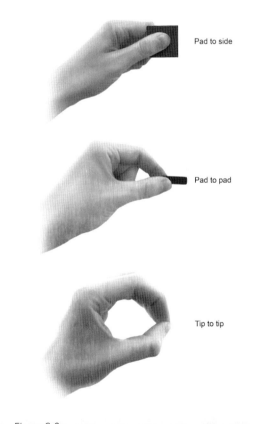

Pad to side

Pad to pad

Tip to tip

Figure 6.3

Types of precision handling

1. In pad-to-side prehension the thumb moves in abduction and adduction without much rotation, so that its pad can reach the side of one of the fingers. It is the least precise form of precision handling, and is used in the action of striking a match.

2. In pad-to-pad prehension the thumb has refined its ability to rotate opposite to the fingers. The pad contacts one of the finger pads, typically the index finger. The thumb is in flexion, abduction, and rotation, and the finger is flexed more in the metacarpophalangeal and proximal interphalangeal joints than in the distal interphalangeal joint. The highest concentration of sensory nerve endings in the body is found in the finger pads, resulting in fine motor control. This is the action of picking up and holding a coin.

3. Tip-to-tip prehension is similar to pad-to-pad prehension, but moves the thumb and finger into greater flexion, so the object is held right at the tip of the fingers rather than on the pad, forming a circle. In the first finger, the position requires adduction at the metacarpalphalangeal joint. This is the action of holding or threading a needle.

Playing with Prehension

Experiment with using a power grip to alternately pick up a cylinder, a small ball, and a suitcase by its handle. How does each grip change the shape of your hand? How does your hand feel, and how does each grip affect the position and movement of your arm, shoulder, and core?

Experiment with precision grip by alternately picking up tiny objects such as needles, beans, and cards with pad-to-pad, tip-to-tip, and pad-to-side grips. How does each grip change your ability to work with the objects? What do the different grips feel like in your hand, and how

do they change the sensation of your arm and shoulder, and even more distant parts of your body?

Pick up a variety of objects, and notice whether you have a tendency to initiate through radial or ulnar deviation. If so, what does it feel like to bring the wrist to a neutral, centered position and perform the same tasks? Bring your awareness to centering your hand through the capitate bone. While maintaining that awareness, can you write with a pen or pencil? Type on a computer or use a mouse? What changes in your mind and the rest of your body?

Weight Bearing on Your Hands

In table position, notice where the weight naturally falls through your hand. Do your hands move toward radial or ulnar deviation?

What happens to your arms and torso when you emphasize weight falling through the ulnar (little finger) side of the hand?

What happens to your arms and torso when you emphasize weight falling through the radial (thumb) side of the hand?

What happens to your arms and torso when you distribute the weight evenly through your hand? With fingers spread or with no space between your fingers?

What happens to your arms and torso when you add a little pressure with the tips of your fingers into the floor, with evenly distributed weight through your palm?

Can you maintain awareness of the palmar arch as weight moves through your hand?

Can you center your weight through the capitate bone?

Embodying the Wrist

The wrist complex is formed by two compound joints, both of which contribute to flexion and extension and to abduction and adduction. The radiocarpal joint is the articulation of the carpus (scaphoid, lunate, and triquetrum) with the radius and its articular disc. The midcarpal joint is an articulation between the proximal and distal carpal rows. The two-joint system permits a large range of motion with minimal articular surfaces within a compact joint capsule. Movement at the wrist complex is necessary for all types of prehension, so lack of movement makes the activities of daily life difficult and places strain at the elbow and shoulder.

The Midcarpal Joint

The compound midcarpal joint has an irregular surface: the distal capitate and hamate form a rounded surface that fits into a socket created by the proximal lunate and triquetrum, while a part of the rounded scaphoid fits into a socket made by the distal trapezoid and trapezium. This arrangement permits sagittal and vertical plane movement but does not permit horizontal rotation.

The Radiocarpal Joint

The radiocarpal joint is formed by the socket of the radius in articulation with a ball formed by the scaphoid, lunate, and triquetrum. The joint is like a ball and socket except that its ovoid shape only permits movement in flexion/extension and adduction/abduction: it does not permit rotation in the horizontal plane. In distal movement of the radiocarpal joint, the proximal carpal bones glide within the concave surface of the radius. In proximal movement the radius travels around the carpals. You can easily feel the scaphoid bone protrude forward during wrist extension and the lunate protrude dorsally during wrist flexion.

Proximal Origination for Distal Movement at the Radiocarpal Joint

Stabilizing your forearm in space, originate movement of the carpals from the articular surface of the radius, as if you were waving goodbye very slowly. Imagine centering the carpals in the joint surface of the radius, and maintain that feeling of centeredness as you move through the entire range of motion. Enjoy the rotation of the carpals in the joint. Explore the sensation as your reach an object or adjust your wrist for other activities such as cooking or typing.

Distal Origination for Proximal Movement at the Radiocarpal Joint

Stabilizing your hand on the floor or another surface, start the movement of the forearm from sensing the articular surface of the carpals. Feel the radius traveling around the carpus. Moving from table position to child's pose, can your carpals support and initiate the movement that flows through your entire body? What happens if you initiate the change from downward to upward facing dog by initiating dorsiflexion of the wrist at the articular surface of the carpals?

The Meniscus

The space between the ulna and the carpal bones is much larger than the articular space between the radius and the carpals. The articular disc occupies part of that space. Distal and medial to the disc is a meniscus, a cartilaginous padding that provides extra resilience and support to the space. It is attached to the pisiform and to the ulnar styloid process. If the pattern of ulnar deviation is strong in the wrist, the meniscus may be condensed. Freeing the meniscus and recovering its resiliency helps to repattern the wrist and to center movement through the capitate bone.

Lubricating the Meniscus

Find the space in your wrist between the styloid process of the ulna and the pisiform bone. Using pad-to-pad prehension, move the tissue between the bones gently to awaken the self-awareness of the cushioning meniscus. If the space feels dry or stiff, use movement to lubricate it—the meniscus can feel like a sponge gradually filling with water. Invite the space to fill completely with a resilient, bouncy sensation and see if it can provide a little stability to your medial wrist. How does that affect your hand and arm?

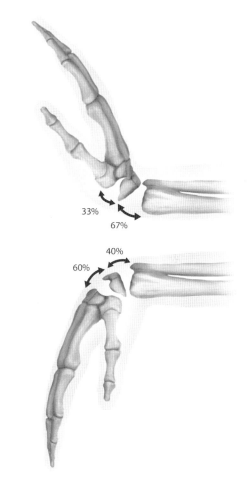

Movement at the Wrist

During flexion of the wrist from neutral, motion begins in the midcarpal joint and is followed by a smaller amount of flexion in the radiocarpal joint (Figure 6.4). During extension of the wrist from neutral, the motion is initated at the radiocarpal with less midcarpal participation. Adduction and abduction also require movement at both joints.

Figure 6.4

Movement at the radioulnar and midcarpal joints

Wrist Flexion and Extension

Surround one wrist with your other hand. Slowly initiate flexion and listen to the internal movement, to feel whether motion at the midcarpal joint precedes motion at the radiocarpal. Notice when your radiocarpal joint begins to move, and where you feel the end of its range of motion. As you let your hand rebound to neutral, notice whether the joints move simultaneously or in sequence.

At neutral once again (neither in flexion or extension) initiate extension at your wrist. Feel whether the radiocarpal joint initiates, when the midcarpal joint joins the movement, and how much movement each articulation contributes to the extension of your wrist. As you let your wrist rebound toward neutral, what is the sequence of joint motion, or is it simultaneous?

Freeing the Wrist Joint

Move a partner's wrist passively through its range of motion in flexion and extension, looking for movement in the radiocarpal and midcarpal joints. Does the movement feel equally free in both directions? Do you sense resistance in one direction? Help your partner's bones to counter rotate and to find space in the joints.

Move the wrist passively through its range of motion in abduction and adduction, feeling for movement both in the radioulnar and midcarpal joints. Does the movement feel equally free in both directions? Is there resistance in either direction? Help your partner's bones to counter rotate and to find space in the joint.

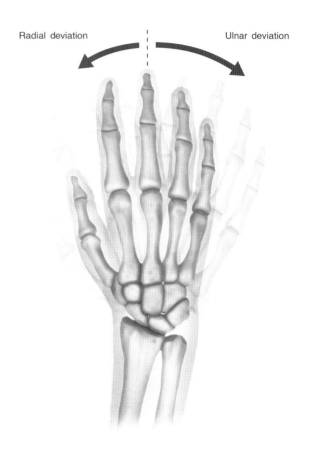

Radial deviation   Ulnar deviation

Figure 6.5

Radial and ulnar deviation

Radial and Ulnar Deviation (Figure 6.5)

In neutral alignment of the wrist and hand, a straight line drawn between the center of the elbow and the center of the wrist would extend through the third finger. Rotation of the hand and forearm occurs through that axis.

Radial deviation is when the hand is positioned or deviates thumb-ward from that line. The space of the scaphoid bone is compressed and the wrist is shortened laterally and lengthened medially. The tilt of the scaphoid allows the trapezium to approach the radius, and the pisiform moves away from the ulna. The space for the articular disc and the meniscus is increased. In supination, radial deviation is normally limited to 15 degrees from straight. In pronation, the angle can be slightly larger.

In ulnar deviation the hand is positioned or deviates toward the little finger. In that case, the triquetrum and pisiform approach the ulna, compressing the space of the meniscus and the articular disc, and the wrist is shortened medially. Ulnar deviation may reach 35 degrees in supination; the

angle can be slightly larger in pronation. In extreme expressions of ulnar deviation the metacarpal and interphalangeal joints may join the deviation in the direction of the little finger.

In neutral alignment the action of the hand is centered on the capitate bone, without deviation to either side, except as is necessary for twisting or rotating an object. Each side of the wrist then has space and freedom for movement, and the wrist has equanimity. While ulnar and radial deviation are necessary components of functional movement, it is helpful to notice whether those tendencies begin to become overemphasized and create problems at the wrist or higher joints.

Radial and Ulnar Deviation

Reach for an object as though you are going to pick it up, and pause just before making contact. What is the position of your wrist? Has it deviated in either abduction or adduction, or have you maintained space on both sides of your wrist? Reach again, this time guiding your hand toward the object from your third finger, feeling equal space on both sides of your wrist. How does your arm feel when you consciously limit ulnar or radial deviation? Play with a series of objects and notice whether their varying shapes influence the degree of deviation in your wrist.

Observation: Radial and Ulnar Deviation

Observe a partner picking up and putting down several objects and gesturing with their hands. Does your partner have a habit of radial or ulnar deviation? Of excess flexion or extension? Does the joint space seem to stay free, or does the meniscus become compressed? Does movement flow down the ulna into the hand? Does movement flow from the radial hand through the radius?

Repatterning Radial and Ulnar Deviation

Once you have noted your partner's habits of movement at the wrist, you may want to support them in establishing more balance. Guide them with touch, helping them to feel space on both sides of the joint as they move toward an object: you may place your hands on both sides of the joint or lead the third finger or capitate bone into space for them. Help your partner notice the moment when the deviation begins, and assist them in slowing down at that point in order to feel the impulse. Help them notice what other joints are affected by the deviation and how they adjust to the new space in the wrist.

Embodying the Forearm

The forearm plays a crucial role in supporting the work of the hand. The two parallel bones of the forearm, the ulna and the radius, articulate with each other at their proximal and distal ends, and form joints with the carpal bones at the wrist and with the humerus at the elbow. If movement at any of the joints at either end of the forearm is restricted, compensations may restrict neighboring joints. The simple act of freeing a restricted forearm can affect the entire body.

The tough connective tissue between the bones—the interosseus membrane—not only maintains the spatial relationship between the bones, but contributes to the strength of the forearm, enabling the two bones to act as one in weight bearing. The fibers are taut when midway between pronation and supination and, in that position, they provide the greatest amount of tensile strength to the forearm.

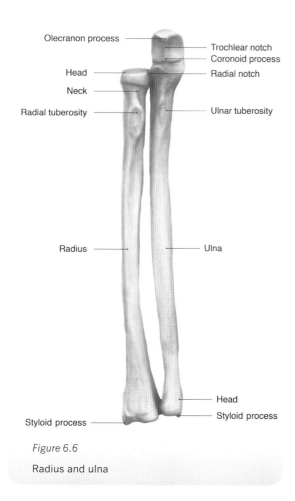

Figure 6.6

Radius and ulna

The Bones and Joints of the Forearm (Figure 6.6)

The Ulna

The ulna is the medial bone of the forearm on the little finger side and may be considered analogous to the tibia in the leg. That analogy holds well at the elbow: the ulna is the primary joint surface with the humerus, just as the tibia is the primary joint surface with the femur at the knee. At the wrist, however, the ulna tapers to a much smaller size relative to the radius, and is not the primary articular bone as is the tibia at the ankle. The ulna's edge can be felt from the elbow to the wrist. The ulna possesses a shaft with a proximal base and a distal

head. Identify and touch (where possible) the following important landmarks on the bone:

Olecranon process

The posterior surface forms the rounded knob of the elbow. Its anterior surface articulates with the humerus and has a small central ridge, the trochlear notch.

Coronoid process

The termination of the articular surface of the ulna's head at the proximal end of the trochlear notch. It is not palpable.

Radial notch

A small concavity lying on the lateral surface of the ulnar head. It articulates with the rounded head of the radius.

The posterior margin

A longitudinal ridge palpable on the posterior surface of the ulna, separating the bone's medial surface from the posterior surface.

The ulnar head

Composed of the articular circumference, the concavity that articulates with the articular disc of the wrist, and the easily palpable styloid process, which projects distally.

Radius

The radius takes its name from a Latin word meaning a spoke of wheel. It is the lateral bone of the forearm, relating to the thumb side of the hand. The radius has a similar role in the forearm to that of the fibula in the leg, supporting mobility. Unlike the fibula's minimal role at the ankle, the radius provides the articular surface at the wrist for the carpus. The proximal head of the radius articulates with both the humerus and the ulna. Identify and touch where possible the following important landmarks on the bone:

Articular fovea

The surface at the proximal end of the radius that articulates with the humerus.

Articular circumference

The band around the head of the radius that rotates on the radial notch of the ulna.

Radial tuberosity

A tuberosity just distal to the head of the radius, on the medial side of the bone.

Carpal articular surface

The concavity at the distal end of the radius that articulates with the carpal bones.

Ulnar notch

The small concavity at the distal end of the bone that receives the articular circumference of the ulna.

Proximal Radioulnar Joint

The proximal radioulnar joint is created by the articulation of the radial notch of the ulna with the articular circumference of the head of the radius. The annular ligament is attached to the ulna and surrounds the articular surface of the radius, which is able to pivot within its embrace.

Distal Radioulnar Joint

The distal radioulnar joint is formed by the head of the ulna and the ulnar notch of the radius. Interposed between the ulna and the carpal bones is the articular disc.

Cellular Respiration: The Forearm

Bring awareness first to your own cellular respiration, emphasizing the breath in your ulna and radius. When your own breathing is well established, share touch with a partner's forearm, maintaining awareness of the underlying skeletal structure. If movement within the tissue arises, follow the movement. If the forearm remains resting, just enjoy the contact!

Mapping the Bones of the Forearm

Map your own or a partner's ulna from the wrist to the elbow. Map the contours of the radius starting at the wrist. Where the overlying muscle makes direct touch difficult, rotate it around the bones, to release the bone from myofascial binding and awaken the periosteum of the underlying bone. Can you palpate the head of the radius within the annular ligament? Can you feel it rotate inside the ligament?

Articular Disc

An articular disc divides a joint space so that each bone at a joint articulates not directly with the neighboring bone, but with the disc interposed between. The articular disc of the wrist, made of fibrocartilagenous connective tissue, plays a role in both the distal radioulnar joint and in the radiocarpal joint. It folds in such a way that it lies between the ulna and the radius, and also extends medially from the radius to continue the joint surface with the carpal bones at the wrist. That part of it occupies the space between the ulna and the carpal bones.

Movement of the Forearm

The rotation of the forearm is called pronation and supination (Figure 6.7). The position of supination is with the palm facing up—as though mimicking a bowl of soup. In that position the bones lie parallel to each other. The movement of pronation brings the palm to face downward, causing the radius to cross over the ulna. Pronation and supination require movement at both the distal and proximal radioulnar joints: moving at one radioulnar joint requires a corresponding movement in the other.

Supination

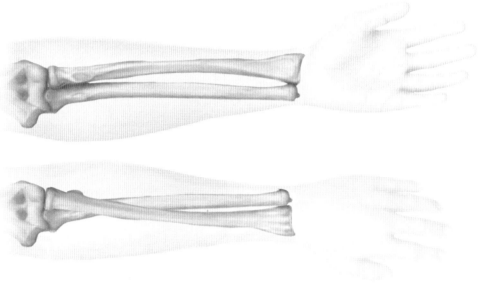

Pronation

Figure 6.7

Pronation and supination

The longitudinal axis of rotation for prona-tion and supination extends from the center of the radial head at the elbow to the center of the ulnar head at the wrist. During rotational move-ment, there is little movement of the proximal ulna. At the distal end, the ulna counters the movement of the radius, moving distally and dor-sally in pronation, and proximally and medially in supination.

Balanced rotation of the forearm is centered from the midpoint of the elbow through the center of the wrist, extending through the third finger. The thumb and little finger rotate simultaneously in opposite directions. If the little finger is stabilized, the thumb and radial hand will arc over the ulnar hand. If the thumb is stabilized, the ulnar hand will rotate under the radial hand.

Forearm Rotation

Holding your forearm with one hand, rotate the other in pronation and supination. Feel the ulna and radius moving under your skin as they cross into pronation and unfold into supination. Feel the difference between the distal portions of the bone and the proximal portions as they move.

- Stabilize your little finger in space as you rotate the radial hand over it.

- Stabilize your thumb in space as you rotate the ulnar hand under it.

- Sense the space between the ulna and radius. Align the rotation through the capi-tate bone and center of the middle finger.

Rotating a Partner's Forearm

Support your partner's forearm by holding the hand and elbow. Use the hand as a lever to alternately pronate and supinate the forearm. If you encounter a feeling of thickness or resistance to rotation in one direction, guide the forearm through its rotational pathway to see if bringing awareness to the bones will increase the range of motion. You may find discontinuity or involuntary motion where there is holding in the nervous system, fascial web, or muscles. If so, decrease the range of motion, go slowly, and encourage your partner to release their bones into gravity as you move them, until you can move through the area of resistance without little movement hiccups. Rotate the forearm around the axes of the thumb, the third finger, and the little finger. When finished with the first arm, invite your partner to notice the difference in sensation between that one and the one that you did not touch.

Touching the Three Layers of Bone

The forearm is a good place to begin working with a partner to differentiate the three layers of bone in touch. You can work with the bones individually or touch them together as one, and practice the ideas for touch and movement presented in Chapter 3.

Sounding into the Forearm

Starting at its distal head, bring your lips to the skin over your radius and vibrate the bone with your voice. Experiment with changing the intensity and pitch of the sound to assess which tone enters the bone tissue most easily. Can the vibration pass through the periosteum into the hard bone and marrow? Move your lips along the surface of your radius toward the elbow, vibrating the entire bone with sound. When finished, notice the difference in sensation between that radius and the other one. If you pronate your arm, you can reach your ulna to do the same thing.

Embodying the Humerus

When we observe the upper arm, we initially tend to notice its muscles, which are much more evident than the underlying structure. The single underlying bone, the humerus, takes its name from the Latin word for shoulder although its participation in the shoulder joint is only one of its functions (Figure 6.8). The humerus has three joints: one with the scapula that forms the shoulder, and two distal joints at the elbow—one with the radius and one with the ulna. Observe the following important landmarks on the bone:

The head of the humerus

The humeral head is a rounded surface that articulates with the scapula. It lies at an angle, proximal and medial to the body of the humerus, with an

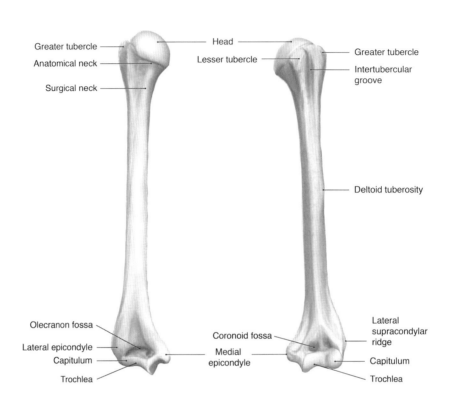

Greater tubercle

Anatomical neck

Surgical neck

Head

Lesser tubercle

Greater tubercle

Intertubercular groove

Deltoid tuberosity

Olecranon fossa

Lateral epicondyle

Capitulum

Trochlea

Coronoid fossa

Medial epicondyle

Lateral supracondylar ridge

Capitulum

Trochlea

Posterior view   Anterior view

Figure 6.8

The left humerus

anatomic neck dividing the smooth articular surface from the rest of the shaft. The head is not palpable.

The greater tubercle

On the lateral side of the bone opposite the head, and usually palpable.

The lesser tubercle

More anterior position than the greater tubercle, close to the head and normally palpable.

The intertubercular sulcus (bicipital groove)

Between the greater and lesser tubercles, and is palpable on most people.

The surgical neck

Just distal to the head and the tubercles.

The deltoid tuberosity

The attachment for the deltoid muscle in the middle of the shaft on the lateral side.

Medial and lateral epicondyles

Palpable protuberances on the sides of the distal end of the humerus, the medial epicondyle larger than the lateral.

Lateral supracondylar ridge

An easily palpable protrusion that leads from the lateral epicondyle proximally toward the midpoint of the shaft. A similar but less palpable ridge lies above the medial epicondyle.

Trochlea

One of two humeral condyles, forms the surface for articulation with the ulna. It has an indented groove, like a waist.

Capitulum

The rounded knob for articulation with the radius.

Olecranon fossa

A pit on the posterior distal surface of the humerus, between the epicondyles, into which the ulnar olecranon process moves during extension of the elbow. It can be felt in some people when the elbow is flexed.

Awakening the Humerus

First map the humeral surfaces that are easily available to your touch, to ensure that the periosteum of the bone feels alive. Then secure the bone at the elbow with one hand while with the other you slide your partner's muscle and fascia horizontally around the humerus. Allow the fascia to stretch and rebound. You are helping your partner's body to differentiate the sensation of bone from the sensation of the muscles.

Cellular Respiration: the Humerus

With a partner, bring your awareness first to your own cellular respiration, emphasizing your humerus. When your own breathing is well established, touch your partner's upper arm, maintaining awareness of the underlying skeletal structure. If movement within the tissue arises, follow the movement. If the arm remains resting, simply enjoy the mutual breathing.

Embodying the Elbow

The elbow is a compound joint having three articulations within the joint capsule: the proximal radioulnar, the humeroradial, and the humeroulnar joints (Figure 6.9). The elbow's ingenious structure allows for rotation between the ulna and radius to occur with ease simultaneously with elbow flexion and extension.

The humeroradial joint is formed by the capitulum of the humerus and the fovea of the proximal radius. It is a ball-and-socket joint, with the radius forming the socket and the humerus forming the ball. In distal movement, the radius travels over the capitulum of the humerus; in proximal movement, the humerus rotates in the socket of the radius. In addition to flexion/extension in the sagittal plane, the radial fovea rotates on the capitulum of the humerus in the horizontal plane, to accommodate pronation and supination.

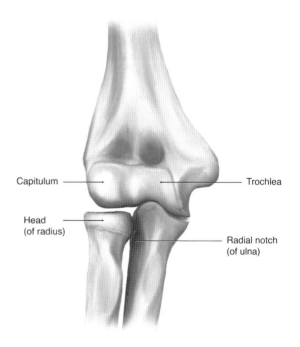

Capitulum — Trochlea

Head (of radius) —

— Radial notch (of ulna)

Figure 6.9

The right elbow, anterior view

The humeroulnar joint is formed by the trochlea of the humerus and the trochlear notch of the ulna. A concave channel in the humeral trochlea guides the leading edge of the ulnar trochlear notch, and limits the movement to flexion and extension through the sagittal plane. In distal movement, the concave ulna travels over the humeral trochlea. In proximal movement, the humerus rotates within the ulnar socket.

The proximal radioulnar joint permits pronation and supination of the forearm, or folding of the radius over the ulna, in conjunction with the distal radioulnar joint. The radial notch is extended by an annular ligament that completely encircles the head of the radius, together forming a ring within which the radial head can pivot.

The angle of the elbow in the sagittal plane, when fully extended, typically reaches 180 degrees in women and 175 degrees in men. The carrying angle is the angle of the fully extended elbow in the vertical plane: it varies between 158 to 180 degrees, with an average of about 168 degrees.

Proximal Initiation of Distal Movement at the Elbow

With the elbow stabilized in space, bring your awareness to the condyles of your humerus. Initiate flexion and extension at the elbow from the condyles. Enjoy space in the joint as the ulna and radius travel over the condylar surfaces. How does the sensation affect your shoulder and your wrist? Can you apply the sensations to movement in daily life?

Distal Initiation of Proximal Movement at the Elbow

From table position place your forearms on the floor to stabilize them. Bring awareness to the trochlear notch of the ulna and the radial fovea. Feeling those surfaces, use them to initiate small movements of the humerus, rocking forward and back in space. Placing your awareness there, notice what happens to the muscles and soft tissues of your arms. How does the movement feel?

Compression and Release of the Elbow

Bring awareness to your partner's elbow by supporting it through its range of motion in flexion/extension and in rotation. Note which directions feel easy and where there might be congestion. Holding the radius near its head and the lateral epicondyle near the capitulum, compress the joint space, and wait for a sense of expansion or rebound. Follow the movement as the bones release away from each other, increasing the joint space.

Supporting the ulna near its proximal end and the medial epicondyle near the trochlea, compress the joint space and wait for a sense of release or rebound. Follow the movement as the bones release away from each other, increasing the joint space. Once again, support your partner's elbow through its range of motion, and see if there is a difference after compression and release.

Embodying the Shoulder Joint

The shoulder (glenohumeral) joint is the articulation between the humeral head and the glenoid fossa of the scapula (Figure 6.10). The head projects medially and superiorly from the shaft of the humerus to meet the scapula. The glenoid fossa is relatively flat and small in relationship to the humeral head. The lack of congruity provides the humerus with a greater range of motion compared to the deep receptacle of the hip joint, but also results in a corresponding decrease in stability. The socket is increased by a labrum, a fibrocartilagenous lip, and supported by a strong ligamentous joint capsule. Because of the relatively unstable skeletal connection, the joint depends on the fascial web, muscles, and the compressive force of gravity to add to its stability.

Because so much of the glenohumeral joint is formed by soft tissue, postural deviations in the shoulder develop easily. Habits of movement can force the humeral head out of a centered relationship with the glenoid fossa. For example, if the anterior muscles that cross the joint become overdeveloped or if the shoulder girdle falls forward, the humeral head can position itself forward in the joint, stressing surrounding tissues and limiting the ease of motion. As we work with movement at the shoulder, it is important to encourage the humeral head to center itself in the glenoid cavity.

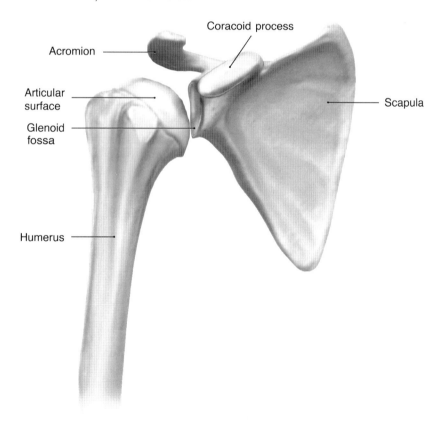

Figure 6.10

The glenohumeral joint

Movement of the Glenohumeral Joint

The glenohumeral joint moves in three degrees of freedom. The following terms are used to describe the motions of the joint:

Flexion

Forward motion of the humerus in the sagittal plane.

Extension

Backward motion of the humerus through the sagittal plane.

Abduction

Motion through the vertical plane away from the center of the body.

Adduction

Motion through the vertical plane toward the center of the body.

Internal rotation

Inward rotation around the longitudinal axis of the arm, in horizontal plane movement.

External rotation

Outward rotation around the longitudinal axis of the arm, in horizontal plane movement.

Horizontal abduction and adduction

Motion that occurs when the arm is elevated at a right angle to the body. The motion of the arm from the side toward midline, maintained at the same level of elevation, is horizontal adduction. Motion of the arm away from midline, maintained at the same level of elevation, is horizontal abduction.

Circumduction

A compound circling movement that occurs when the humerus maps the surface of a cone, with the tip of the cone at the shoulder joint.

Centering the Joint

From the side, observe the positioning of a partner's shoulder joint. Independent of the shoulder girdle, does the joint itself appear to roll forward, to be held up from the neck, or to be thrust back? When the partner moves to supine, does the joint retain its position?

With your partner either supine or sitting, compress the humeral head into the glenoid fossa. Use the release to encourage a sense of congruence and space within the joint. Encourage your partner's humeral head to sense the entire surface of the glenoid fossa.

You may want to release the humerus and shoulder area from myofascial binding before you repeat the compression and release. It may be helpful to change position as well. Support the surrounding tissues to become mobile, so that the humeral head can center itself in the joint.

Counter Rotation at the Shoulder

Any distal movement of the humerus (and, by extension, the whole arm) produces a countermovement of the scapula. When the hand and humerus move sagitally forward the inferior angle of the scapula will move sagitally back. When the hand and humerus move sagitally back the inferior angle of the scapula will press forward into the torso. When the hand and humerus move into abduction, the first movement of the scapula will be the approach of the inferior angle toward the spine. When the hand and humerus move toward midline, the inferior angle will travel laterally. If the humerus rotates medially, the medial border of the scapula moves into the ribs. If the humerus rotates laterally, the medial border releases toward the back.

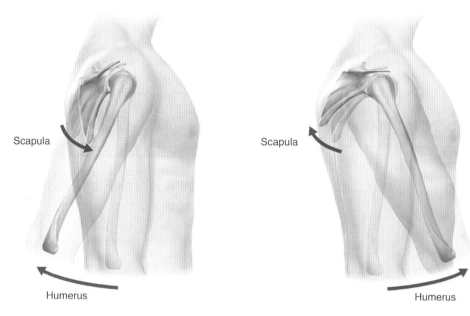

Figure 6.11

Counter rotation at the glenohumeral joint

Counter Rotation at the Glenohumeral Joint (Fig 6.11)

Place one hand on a partner's humerus and the other hand on the inferior angle of the scapula. Invite movement of your partner's arm in flexion and extension, in adduction and in abduction, in internal and external rotation, and in circumduction. Do you feel a counter rotation between the humerus and the scapula? If not, can you facilitate the counter rotation so that the scapula is free to move?

Embodying the Shoulder Girdle

The shoulder girdle is composed of the two shoulder blades and the two collarbones (clavicles)

(Figure 6.12). The shoulder girdle is the foundation for movement of the arms and hands, in much the same way that the pelvis forms the foundation for movement of the legs and feet. In contrast to the fairly rigid pelvis, the shoulder girdle is characterized by a great deal of mobility and allows more spatially complex and expressive movement.

The shoulder girdle does not articulate directly with the spine in the way the pelvis does. Compare the shoulder girdle's skeletal pathway with the directness and immediacy of the sacrum-to-ilium-to-femur articulations in the lower extremities. The articular pathway from spine to humerus follows the forward curve of the ribs from the vertebral segments to the sternum; from the sternum to the clavicles; from there to the scapulae; and finally into the humerus at the glenohumeral joints. By this arrangement, the arms are less tethered to the central axis and enjoy greater freedom of movement and more spatial choices. But it is

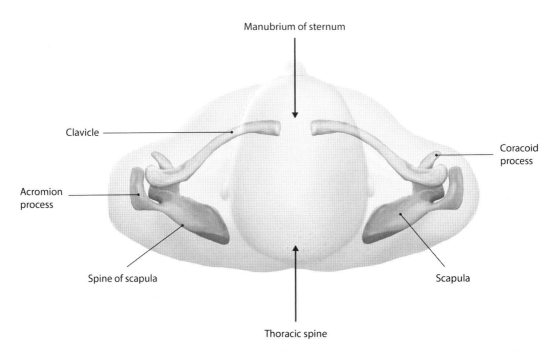

Manubrium of sternum

Clavicle

Coracoid process

Acromion process

Spine of scapula

Scapula

Thoracic spine

Figure 6.12

Shoulder girdle

important to note that indirect does not mean weak. There is a great deal of power in the upper extremities, due to the muscular, ligamentous, and fascial architecture of the system. While the hands, arms, and shoulders can support our body weight on the ground, they also allow brachiation, monkey-like overhead locomotion from one handhold to another.

Remember that the shoulder girdle can be an area of emotional holding. As you work with students or partners in hands-on skeletal applications, be particularly aware of changes in their breathing, tone, communication, and awareness. Those changes may indicate that an emotional or energetic release is accompanying the physical change. Stay in dialogue and support your partner in a spacious way. Do not force the changes to either stop or continue and do not go beyond what is comfortable for both of you.

The Bones of the Shoulder Girdle

The Scapula

The scapula is an elegantly organized bone positioned over the second to seventh ribs (Figure 6.13). Once again, the themes of stability and mobility arise in the shape of the bone itself, with the large flattish blade supporting the stability of the upper extremities, and the knobby, complex superior and anterior portions presenting many surfaces for muscular and ligamentous attachments to permit movement. The large triangular blade looks flat, but is actually slightly curved to slide over the ribs of the superior and lateral back.

The triangular shape of the human scapula is more delicate and mobile than the quadrilateral scapula of lower primates and other mammals whose forequarters are utilized for consistent weight bearing. This triangular shape facilitates the important rotary action of the scapula, in

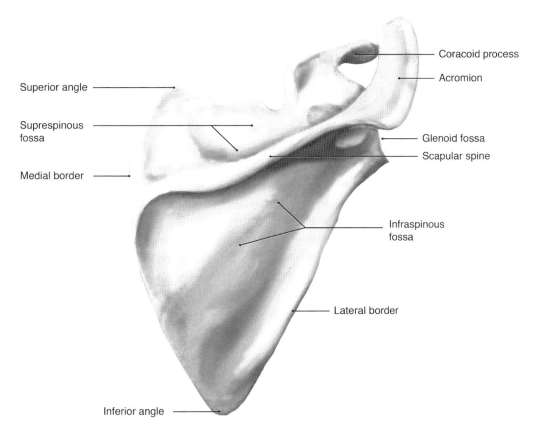

Figure 6.13

The scapula

which the superior angle, inferior angle, and gle-noid fossa counterbalance each other in rotating around a fulcrum near the center of the blade. If any of those points fail to move freely, movement of the arm and back will be constricted. Identify the following:

Acromion

The portion that overhangs and protects the shoulder joint.

Glenoid fossa

Lateral-facing socket that forms the scapular portion of the shoulder joint (in Greek, glene

means joint socket and eidos means resemblance). The glenoid fossa is aptly named, since it resembles a joint socket but is flat, and not fully formed.

Coracoid process

A beak-like tip that projects forward to the front of the body, palpable just beneath the lateral portion of the clavicle.

Spine of the scapula

The easily palpable posterior ridge from the acromion to the medial border that separates the supraspinous and infraspinous fossae.

Supraspinous fossa

The depression above the spine of the scapula

Infraspinous fossa

The depression below the spine of the scapula.

Medial border

The length of the blade that lies adjacent to the spine.

Lateral border

The side of the blade that lies beneath the armpit.

Superior angle

The sharp corner at the top of the medial border.

Inferior angle

The lower tip of the scapula, where the medial border meets the lateral border.

Subscapular fossa

The concave depression located on the anterior surface of the scapular blade.

Scapular Holding

This is a very simple and supportive way to bring awareness to the scapulae. With your partner lying supine, sitting at their head, simply place your hands symmetrically underneath the scapulae. Invite your partner to release their bones and breathe into your receptive hands. Follow movement if any arises. Feel your partner's breath.

The Clavicle

The clavicle is the slender S-shaped collarbone that connects the sternum with the shoulder blade. The most frequently broken bones in the human body, the clavicles lie just under the skin like wings coming off the top of the sternum, and can be seen and felt easily in most people. They support the shoulder, acting like struts that align the shoulders on the ribs. In birds, the two clavicles are centrally joined, forming the wishbone that provides stability for the thorax in flight. The clavicle is anteriorly convex in the medial two-thirds of its length, and anteriorly concave in its lateral portion. The end at the acromioclavicular joint is flattened, and the sternal end is rounded.

A thorough mapping of the scapula and clavicle is a great entry point for working with the shoulder girdle. Mapping them in an upright sitting position emphasizes active weight-flow through the shoulder girdle. Mapping them in sidelying emphasizes release and relaxation. Both positions are helpful.

Mapping the Shoulder Girdle

Begin touch at the broad and easily palpated acromion process. From the posterior acromion find the spine of the scapula and trace it to the medial border. Reaching the medial border, walk your fingers up to the superior angle and down toward the inferior angle. At the medial border you may choose to elevate and slightly retract your partner's shoulder joint: in this position, you can access the undersurface of the scapula, adjusting your quality of touch in order to dive gently under the muscular attachments. You may want to use the inferior angle as a lever to introduce movement, sliding the scapula over the ribs. Walk your fingers up the lateral border as far as you can. At a certain point the bone disappears beneath muscle, but in some individuals you can map the bone very close to the glenoid fossa. Bringing your fingers back to the acromion, find the prominence of the acromioclavicular joint. From there map the clavicle toward the sternum and find the sternoclavicular joint. Mobilize the joint by lifting and moving your partner's shoulder. Walking your fingers back to the acromioclavicular joint, feel beneath the clavicle at that point and see if you can identify the small promontory of the coracoid process. It can be a tender site, so be gentle. You will know if you have found it by pressing it toward the back of the body. If the blade of the scapula in back moves, you know you have found it!

Invite your partner to compare the side that has been mapped to the one that has not. How does it feel, and how does it move?

Resting the Shoulder Girdle

We can minimize tension in the upper body by resting the shoulder girdle on the ribs, rather than having it hang from its muscular and fascial connections to the neck. Imagine the scapula and clavicle as a ring and the ribs as a cone. When the ring is perfectly balanced on the cone, the arms receive support from below. If the ring tilts off the horizontal in any direction or if the shoulder girdle is held in an elevated position, muscular compensation is required and additional stresses are loaded onto the body's structure to maintain equilibrium. That can result in physical limitation or pain within the shoulder girdle or at a distant point in the body.

Resting the Shoulder Girdle

On yourself or a partner, map the ring that is formed by the two clavicles and the scapular spines. Imagine in standing that the ring is parallel to the surface of the earth. Release your head forward as far as you can go without disturbing the horizontal organization of the ring: you may be surprised how little movement is available! Repeat to the back and sides. Then tip the edges of the ring to the front, back, and sides, allowing the head to fall in that direction. Rather than rising from your head, recover your verticality by encouraging the ring to reposition itself in

its horizontal relationship to the earth. The head should float into position.

Now sense the dome of your ribs: wide at the bottom and narrow at the top—perhaps touching them at their widest and again under the armpits where they narrow. Invite the ring of the shoulder girdle to rest evenly and horizontally on that support.

Can your arms relax from the support of the ribs? Can your neck and head float above, independent from the arms and shoulders? Invite movement of your arms in space and maintain the sensation that the shoulder girdle is resting on the ribs.

The Scapulothoracic Joint

The scapulothoracic joint is the articulation of the anterior scapular surface with the ribs. It is not a true joint, since it lacks a capsule, but experientially it is helpful to treat the articulation as a joint. The sliding movement of the scapula on the thorax occurs in relationship to the movements at the acromioclavicular and the sternoclavicular joints.

Movement of the Scapulothoracic Joint

From its resting position, the scapula moves in six basic directions. Most actions of the shoulder and arm utilize combinations of those movements. The following specialized terms are used to describe the basic movements of the scapula:

Elevation

The scapula slides across the ribs upward toward the head.

Depression

The scapula slides across the ribs downward toward the tail.

Abduction

The scapula slides laterally away from the spine.

Adduction

The scapula slides medially toward the spine.

Upward rotation

The inferior angle moves laterally away from the spine, while the superior angle moves toward the spine.

Downward rotation

The inferior angle moves medially toward the spine, while the superior angle moves away from the spine.

Scapular winging

The medial border of the scapula displaces in a posterior direction and the lateral border moves anteriorly. This motion helps to maintain close contact of the scapula with the thorax.

Scapular tipping

The inferior angle moves in a posterior direction and the coracoid process moves in a forward direction. This motion helps to maintain close contact of the scapula with the thorax.

Moving the Shoulder Girdle

Elevate your scapulae, bringing your shoulders toward your ears, and hold the position for a moment. What emotional, gestural, or postural meaning does the position evoke for you?

Depress your scapulae forcefully, downward toward your tail. Hold that position for a moment, and feel its significance as a gesture or posture.

Abduct your scapulae, sliding them laterally, away from the spine. How does this feel, and what resonates with you in the posture?

Slide your scapulae medially in adduction, toward your spine, and hold them in that position. What is the expressive significance of this position, and how does it resonate in your emotions and mind?

Lift one arm above your head, and feel the upward rotation of the scapula as the inferior angle slides laterally toward your armpit. Can you feel the movement and allow the scapula to support the elevated arm? Do the same with the other arm and compare the sensations.

Bringing an arm down to resting from an elevated position, feel the inferior angle of the scapula move medially toward the spine. Can you sense the change in its position?

Finally combine all of these motions to allow the shoulder blades to ride freely over your ribs. Enjoy movement initiated in the shoulder girdle and let it flow from there into your arms and hands.

Shoulder Girdle Mobilization

With your partner lying in front of you on their left side, position yourself so that you can place your right hand on the anterior shoulder and clavicle and left hand on the scapula. Gently move the shoulder girdle in elevation/depression and abduction/adduction. If there is resistance from the soft tissues go slowly and encourage movement to be smooth and continuous, improvising changes of direction and speed. Add the movement of upward and downward rotation by shifting your right hand to the arm and moving it to allow the scapula to rotate. Gradually increase the scale of the movement to include the ribs and spine. When finished, invite your partner to notice the difference between their right and left shoulders. Repeat on the other side.

Weight Bearing on the Arms

In a simple plank or table position, or even with hands against a wall, can you maintain easy and even support of the shoulder girdle, with space in each joint and width between the scapulae? Experiment with some other weight-bearing positions, such as downward facing dog or handstand, and see how your scapulae respond to the change of position. Do they tend to wing, adduct, or abduct excessively in any of those positions?

The Acromioclavicular Joint

The meeting point of the scapula and the clavicle, the acromioclavicular joint is a synovial joint with three degrees of freedom. The lateral end of the clavicle has a small convex facet that joins with the small concave facet of the acromion of the scapula. Because of its irregular surfaces, however, the joint is considered incongruent and there is considerable individual variation in the angle of the joint. Through two years of age, the joint is actually a fibrocartilagenous union. Eventually, a joint space develops, and the remaining fibrocartilage may develop into a disc within the joint. The disc often degenerates in middle age and the joint space typically narrows again by the sixth decade of life.

Movement of the Acromioclavicular Joint

The acromioclavicular joint has a small amount of movement in three directions, which are synonymous with the associated motions of the scapula.

Rotation

The primary movement of the acromioclavicular joint, the joint rotates around a sagittal axis. It is synonymous with the rotation of the scapula on the scapulothoracic joint.

Winging

Winging occurs around a vertical axis, allowing the medial border of the scapula to displace in a posterior direction, and the lateral border to displace anteriorly. Winging at the acromioclavicular joint can be habitual and pathological or a response to scapular abduction and adduction, when the scapula slides around the contour of the ribcage.

Tipping

In tipping, in the joint rotates around the horizontal axis, which produces posterior displacement of the inferior angle and anterior movement of the superior border of the scapula.

The Sternoclavicular Joint

The sternoclavicular joint, which joins the sternum with the clavicle, is the foundation of the shoulder girdle, since it is the bony connection of the shoulder girdle into the trunk. It is a complex incongruent joint. An articular disc between the two bones provides cushioning, fills the incongruity of the joint, and provides a pivot for the movement of the joint. The superior portion of the clavicular head does not articulate with the sternum, but is an attachment site for the articular disc and several ligaments.

Movement of the Sternoclavicular Joint

The sternoclavicular joint has three degrees of freedom (Figure 6.14). Because the bone lies perpendicular to the longitudinal axis of the body, the motions are difficult to define traditionally, and have specialized terminology. The motions at the sternoclavicular joint are defined by the direction of the acromial end of the bone:

Elevation

The clavicle rises headward.

Depression

The clavicle descends tailward.

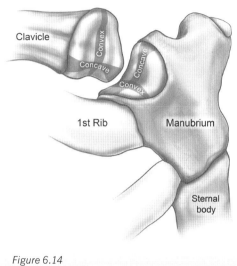

Figure 6.14

Sternoclavicular joint

Protraction

The clavicle moves forward of the vertical plane.

Retraction

The clavicle moves dorsally.

Rotation

The clavicle rotates in either direction around its longitudinal axis.

Both bones, the clavicle and the manubrium, offer saddle-shaped surfaces, so that each bone is able to alternate between the roles of ball and socket. In elevation and depression, the rounded inferior surface of the clavicle is a ball that rotates in the shallow socket of the manubrium. The articular disc forms a unit with the manubrium, and the clavicle rotates within this disc-manubrium complex. In protraction and retraction, the bones switch roles, and the rounded aspect of the manubrium rotates within the concavity of the clavicular head. In this case, the articular disc forms a unit with the clavicle, and the manubrium rotates within the disc-clavicle complex.

In many people, the clavicular joint spaces become compressed as a result of forward rounding of the shoulders. If the rotator cuff muscles hold excess tension, the joint space in the shoulder can be compressed as well. By helping your partner open the joint spaces, the shoulder girdle can take its place easily on top of the ribs.

Encouraging Space

Sternoclavicular Joint

Identify and map the articulation and gently place your hand or fingers above it. Ask your partner to breathe into the space of the joint. With one hand on the sternum and the other on the clavicle, compress and release the joint. Invite your partner to imagine a spring emerging from the center of the joint, allowing water to flow along the clavicle and widen into the shoulder joint.

Acromioclavicular Joint

Identify and map the articulation, and gently place your hand or fingers above it. Invite your partner to breathe into the space of the joint. With one hand on the acromion and the other on the clavicle, compress and release the joint. Again, invite your partner to imagine and feel water flowing from the joint, across the head of the humerus and into the floor. Invite them to notice any sensations that may emerge in other parts of the body.

Glenohumeral Joint

Find the joint beneath the acromion of the scapula. Invite your partner to breathe into the joint space. Placing one hand on the humeral head and the other on the scapula, compress and release the joint. Invite the joint space to expand in two directions—toward the arm and toward the shoulder girdle. It might help to imagine the bubbles in a fish tank emerging from the center of the joint.

After working with each joint on one side, invite your partner to move their arm, and notice the difference between that side and the one that has not been touched.

Sequencing Compression Through the Shoulder Girdle

With your partner supine or sitting, hold the humerus. Find a pathway from the humerus to the sternum, compressing the humerus into the glenoid fossa, following into the acromioclavicular and sternoclavicular joints.

Find a posterior pathway toward the spine, compressing the humerus into the glenoid fossa and sequencing the compression into the scapulothoracic joint and then toward the spine.

Find a central pathway, allowing the compression of the shoulder joint to flow equally through the anterior and posterior pathways.

Scapulohumeral Rhythm

Scapulohumeral rhythm is the combination and sequencing of movement at the scapulothoracic, glenohumeral, acromioclavicular, and sternoclavicular joints in the action of lifting the arm overhead (Figure 6.15). From its resting place hanging into gravity, the arm normally has a range of 180 degrees, allowing it to rise vertically toward the sky through flexion or abduction. While there are many individual variations, the movement of the scapula over the ribs normally contributes 60 degrees of motion, and the glenohumeral joint contributes 120 degrees of motion (Levangie, 2011). There are several advantages to that arrangement:

- The distribution of action permits a larger range of motion with less compromise of stability than if a similar range were permitted at a single joint.

- The movement of the scapula allows the humeral head to remain in optimal contact with the glenoid fossa, reducing the shearing forces that would occur with movement at only one joint.

- The movement at multiple joints permits the muscles acting on the glenohumeral joint to work within a more contained and productive length-to-tension ratio.

Scapulohumeral rhythm requires coordinated movement at the sternoclavicular and acromioclavicular joints in addition to the scapulothoracic joint to facilitate the rotation of the scapula. The first 30 degrees of motion occur through clavicular elevation at the sternoclavicular joint, which moves around a sagittal axis that pierces both the joint and the spine of the scapula at the medial border.

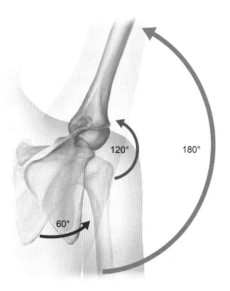

120°   180°

60°

Figure 6.15

Scapulohumeral rhythm

3. Between 90 degrees and 120 degrees of arm elevation, the scapula continues to rotate on the thorax, with movement primarily at the acromioclavicular joint.

4. Between 120 degrees and 180 degrees of arm elevation, movement occurs again primarily in the glenohumeral joint as the scapula stabilizes the movement.

Exploring Scapulohumeral Rhythm

With a partner or by yourself, touch your sternoclavicular joint with the opposite hand and raise your arm overhead. Feel when and how movement occurs at the joint. How closely does it match the model presented above?

Touch your acromioclavicular joint with the opposite hand, and raise your arm overhead. Feel when and how movement occurs at the joint. How closely does it match the model?

Stabilize your scapula and move your arm at the glenohumeral joint as far as you can without moving the scapula or the clavicle. How large is your range of motion? How closely does it match the model?

Initiate movement of the shoulder girdle by sliding the scapula in every direction against the ribs. Notice what motions are required at the acromioclavicular and sternoclavicular joints as you move. Then move your arm freely in space, and feel the contribution of each joint and the sliding of the scapula. Initiate movement from the scapula into the arms, and then from the fingers into the scapula.

Repeat all the steps above while bearing weight on your arms, and notice what is different.

The last 30 degrees of scapular rotation occur on a sagittal axis at the acromioclavicular joint; the clavicle stabilizes at the end of its range of motion, and the scapula continues its upward rotation through movement at the acromioclavicular joint.

Scapulohumeral rhythm helps us to understand the contribution of each joint. While your movement is likely to differ a bit from the model, it is likely that if movement is restricted at any of the contributing joints, the range of movement in the arm will be diminished. Here is the model of how joints work together to raise the arm to 180 degrees:

1. The first 60 degrees of arm elevation occur primarily in the glenohumeral joint with the scapula stabilized against the thorax.

2. Between 60 degrees and 90 degrees of arm elevation, the scapula begins its first 30 degrees of upward rotation, with the movement primarily in the sternoclavicular joint.

Embodying the Ribs and Sternum

The ribs and sternum are the structural support for the shoulder girdle and arms. When the arms move freely, the root of their movement is in the thorax. With its 88 joints and 27 spiraling bones, the structure is ready to accommodate the rise and fall of breath, the motion of the rotating spine, and the pull of a lifting arm—and to perform all of those motions at the same time. The ribs and sternum adapt to infinite variations of posture and use, while protecting our internal organs.

The English language calls this complex of bones and joints a ribcage. Emphasizing the cage-like aspect of the structure is unfortunate, because the term undermines its marvelous mobility. The word rib derives from an Old English word meaning to roof over: the image of ribs forming a roof over the heart seems much more warming and less restrictive than that of a cage. The word ribcage is used in this text, but with the understanding that it does not have to contain the breath, restrict the energetic flow of the heart, or keep us imprisoned in any way.

The fundamental movement of the ribs and sternum is breath, creating space for the expanding and condensing rhythm of the lungs. There are many styles of breathing, and many techniques that purport to teach us how to breathe. The fact is that we can adapt to an infinite number of breath patterns, and each of us has an individuated way of breathing that serves our needs. That said, skeletal embodiment of the ribs and sternum can give us more pleasure and ease in breathing.

The Sternum

The sternum consists of three flat bones forming the frontal attachment for the ribs (Figure 6.16).

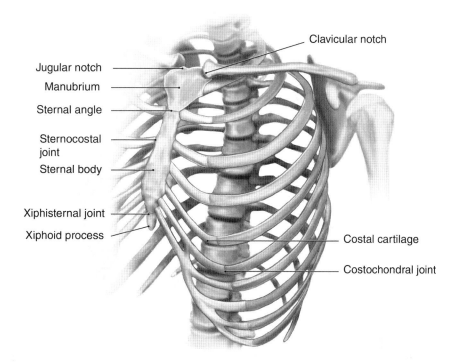

Jugular notch
Manubrium
Sternal angle
Sternocostal joint
Sternal body
Xiphisternal joint
Xiphoid process

Clavicular notch

Costal cartilage
Costochondral joint

Figure 6.16

The sternum

Seen from the side, it resembles a curved dagger, with a sharp inferior tip and a widened and curved superior portion. The sternum protects several frontal structures of the chest cavity, including the heart, thymus gland, and portions of the lungs, as well as deeper structures such as the trachea, esophagus, and aorta.

Manubrium

The superior bone of the sternum, the manubrium is shaped something like a Greek cross. At the cranial end of the bone is the jugular notch, the bony depression at the base of the throat, and lateral to that are the clavicular notches, providing the articulating surface with the clavicles. Close to the clavicular notches are the paired costal notches, forming joints with the first ribs.

Sternal Body

The sternal body is elongated, slightly narrower at the top than at the bottom, and forms the bulk of the sternum, lying directly over the heart. Its borders have symmetrical costal notches for the attachments of the third through seventh ribs.

The Sternal Angle

The sternal angle is the joint between the manubrium and the sternal body: the angle between the bones is about 140 degrees. Designed to accommodate the motion of breath with movement in the sagittal plane, it originates as a synchondrosis that develops into a symphysis, similar in design to the symphysis pubis. In some people, the central portion of the disc can disappear to create a synovial joint space. In others, primarily older adults, the joint ossifies, probably due to lack of use.

Locating the sternal angle on yourself provides important reference points for other structures. The second ribs project from the angle, allowing you to count your ribs from that point. It also marks the level of the fifth thoracic vertebral segment and the point of bifurcation of the trachea into the bronchi of the lungs.

Locating the Sternal Angle

If you move your fingers down from the center of your neck, they will land on the superior bony surface of your sternum: the jugular notch of the manubrium. Slowly move your fingers down the surface of the manubrium, mapping the periosteum. Very soon your fingers will come upon a horizontal bump or protrusion, about three fingers wide. That bump is your sternal angle: above the bump is the manubrium, below is the sternal body. If you walk your fingers horizontally you will be able to palpate your second rib.

With the fingers of one hand on your manubrium and other on your sternal body, invite a series of breaths high into your lungs and chest. Do you feel movement at that joint? If not, simply imagine that the sternal body rises from the manubrium with your inhalation and descends with your exhalation.

The Xiphoid Process

The xiphoid process is named for the Greek word for sword, which it resembles in its sharply tapered point. Based on patterns of use, the xiphoid is quite variable in shape: it may be forked, have a foramen, or be twisted or bent. It is the anterior attachment for the breathing diaphragm and is a site of attachment for ligaments and muscles at the center of the body.

The Xiphisternal Joint

The xiphisternal joint is a synchondrosis joining the sternal body and the xiphoid process, which may ossify by 40 to 50 years of age. The costal notch for the seventh rib sometimes articulates with the xiphisternal joint as well. Like the sternal angle, it is designed to move in the sagittal plane with the motion of breath: the distal tip of the xiphoid process moves forward with exhalation as the diaphragm and torso expand and back toward the center of the body with exhalation. Many of us suffer from reversed breath patterns: the xiphoid process may not move at all (leading to ossification of the joint) or it may be sucked inward with inhalation and forced forward with exhalation. In an infant's first breath, it will expand forward if there is ease, but if the breath emerges as part of a startle response, the xiphoid contracts toward the back of the body, establishing a reversed breathing pattern. It is helpful to explore the mobility of the xiphoid process in breathing, allowing it to expand outward with the inhalation and return to resting upon exhalation.

Breath and the Xiphoid Process

Lying supine, with knees elevated and feet on the floor, take a few breaths to settle your mind and body. Imagine that you are breathing through a straw in your navel center. Your belly will float toward the ceiling with inhalation and settle down to rest with your exhalation.

Place one hand above your xiphoid process. Can you feel the joint and the bone, or are they hidden? Can you feel the bone's movement, or is it fixed in space? Whatever your experience is, imagine that within your abdominal inhalation the tip of your xiphoid process elevates toward the ceiling and with your exhalation it falls with your navel back toward the center.

Does this change the sensation of your breath pattern? Does it alter the movement of your ribs? How do you feel, physically, mentally, and emotionally as you embody this part of yourself?

The Ribs

Each of the 12 thoracic vertebral segments supports a pair of ribs that sweep around to the front of the body, encircling the chest cavity (Figure 6.17). There is a spiraling three-dimensional complexity to the shape of the ribs: in addition to their curving surfaces, most

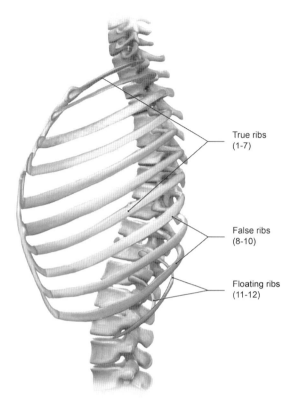

True ribs (1-7)

False ribs (8-10)

Floating ribs (11-12)

Figure 6.17

The ribs

ribs also twist along their longitudinal axis. Each of your 24 ribs has a head, a neck, and a body. The first rib is widened through its body, and sits closer to the horizontal plane, forming a table-like structure for the support of the neck and head. From the second rib on, each successive rib's angle of descent from back to front increases slightly so that the rib ends at a much lower position than its head's origin. From the sixth through tenth ribs, this arrangement forces the costal cartilage to travel upward to join the sternum. The eleventh and twelfth ribs articulate only with the spine, with free distal ends. Rarely, some people may have additional cervical or lumbar ribs or only eleven pairs in the thoracic area.

Together the ribs form a dome—an ovoid shape from the width of the mid-chest, narrowing sharply upward under the shoulders to the small first ribs. The top of the dome supports the ring of the shoulder girdle.

Reach of the Hand Supported by the Ribs

Lift one arm to 90 degrees in front of you with immobilized ribs, and notice the distance that the arm can reach. Placing your other hand at one of your highest ribs, allow that rib to move forward in space, feeling the resulting forward shift of the hand in space. Do the same thing in succession down the ribs, and notice how releasing each rib increases the spatial reach of the hand.

Do the same experiment lifting the arm overhead. Reach your hand up to the sky without allowing the ribs to join the movement. Then allow the ribs of that side to elongate and support the length of the arm. Which movement do you prefer? How does it feel to allow the movement of your arms to start in your ribs?

True Ribs

The first through seventh ribs are called the true ribs, because they articulate directly with the sternum.

False Ribs

The eighth through 10th ribs are called false ribs, because their cartilaginous attachments join into a common insertion at the base of the sternal body.

Floating Ribs

The 11th and 12th ribs articulate only with the spine so are called floating ribs: their extremities have no articulation.

A complete mapping of the ribs is a wonderful experience for the receiver and invaluable for the active partner in understanding the dynamic sweep of the ribs from back to front. The mapping itself will assist rib

mobility and provide a sense of dimensionality in the chest. However, as we utilize touch to stimulate awareness, we need to remember that the closer we get to the center of the body, the more touch may elicit emotions and personal sensitivities. As you work with a partner's ribs in hands-on applications of the material, be particularly aware of changes in your partner's breathing, tone, communication, and awareness. Those changes may indicate emotional release accompanying physical change. Observation of breath and changing tone in the body and mind will give you clues to your partner's experience and needs. As you work with the sternum and the ribs, it is particularly important to make agreements about appropriate touch.

Mapping the Ribs

Work with your partner in sidelying, facing away from you. Ask your partner to help you locate the xiphoid process: From there you can locate the 10th rib and map it with periosteal touch from front to back. Return to the bottom of the sternum to find the ninth rib, and do the same thing. Work up the ribs in sequence on that side.

Make that you are both comfortable with touching and being touched around the sensitive areas; if your partner is female she may want to shift her breast tissue out of the way or not be mapped in that area. The seventh through second ribs will be partly covered by the scapula: do your best to connect the anterior with the spinal portions of those ribs. Moving the arm to rotate the scapula can provide a little more access. Most importantly, remember that you do not need to be perfect. On some people it is easy to map the ribs and on others muscles and other tissue obscure their location. Enjoy the process—your partner will feel the results either way.

When finished, be sure to check with your partner and listen to what their experience was in this exploration.

Variations on Mapping the Ribs

Rocking Variation

Identify and hold an individual rib on the front of your partner's body and higher up on the back of the body. Increasing your pressure on one side, feel for movement at the other side. If movement is free, rock the rib gently back and forth, and repeat at neighboring ribs.

Cradling the Floating Ribs

With your partner in prone position, cradle the floating ribs by placing your palms on the trunk directly over them. Invite breath into your hand and suggest that the ribs can float away toward the ceiling while the breath comes into your hand. Try placing one finger at the costovertebral joint and one finger above the end of the rib, and invite the space between them to fill with breath.

Costovertebral Joints

The articulations that join most ribs to the spine are the costovertebral joints. At the head of each rib, one articular facet articulates with the vertebra above and another articulates with the numerically corresponding segment below. Between these vertebral articulations, the surface of the head also communicates with the intervertebral disc. This triad of joints is enclosed within a single joint capsule. In addition to the movement of breath, each rib therefore responds to the spatial movement of two vertebral segments and their interposed disc. The motion at those joints consists of rotation and gliding (Figure 6.18). This arrangement holds true for ribs two through nine: the first, tenth, eleventh, and twelfth ribs articulate with only their own vertebral segments.

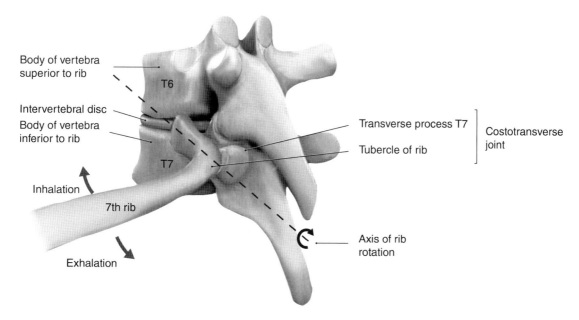

Body of vertebra superior to rib

T6

Intervertebral disc

Body of vertebra inferior to rib

Transverse process T7

Tubercle of rib

Costotransverse joint

T7

Inhalation

7th rib

Exhalation

Axis of rib rotation

Figure 6.18

Rotation at costovertebral and costotransverse joints

Compression and Release of the Costovertebral Joints

This requires a little patience, a little, imagination, and some confidence, because it can be difficult to locate the joints between the ribs and the vertebral bodies. The actual joint is buried within muscles and ligaments, but once you find a rhythm it can be deeply satisfying for your partner.

With your partner prone or in side lying, find the upward direction of one of the lower ribs as it approaches the spine. Using the fingers of one hand, find a comfortable hold on the rib and visualize the points of contact of the rib with two vertebral bodies. With your other hand find a point of leverage on the adjacent spinous process or the opposite side of the spine to move the spine toward the rib while you encourage the rib to move toward the spine. Compress and release.

Repeat the process in as many costovertebral joints as you can. When complete, invite your partner to sit or stand and move, sensing any differences in the ribs, spine, or surrounding tissues.

Costotransverse Joints

At the meeting point between the neck and the body of each rib lies a tubercle. From vertebrae T-1 through T-7, there is a synovial joint between each rib's tubercle and a concave pit (fovea) on the transverse process of its numerically corresponding vertebra. The resulting costotransverse joint allows the rib to rotate within the socket of the transverse process. From T-8 through T-10, the articular surfaces become flattened, and the movement shifts from rotation to gliding. The costovertebral is superior to the costotransverse joint, and motion at the two joints must be reciprocal. The floating ribs at T-11 and T-12 have no costotransverse joints.

Lateral Flexion from the Ribs

Standing comfortably, bend your torso to one side, and then return to the vertical. To the best of your abilities, limit movement to the vertical plane, without rotation or flexion/extension.

Repeat the movement but this time visualize air moving through the spaces between your ribs. As your body bends to the side, feel the spaces on that side diminishing, while the spaces between the ribs on the opposite side expand, allowing more air to pass through. Guide the movement by balancing the sense of the expanding space with that of the decreasing space on the other side and observe how it influences the movement. Return to vertical reversing the process; decrease the spaces between ribs on your lengthened side and increase the spaces on your shortened side.

Costal Cartilage

The rib does not articulate directly with the sternum: it is connected by a cartilaginous extension that completes the arc of the rib to the front of the body. The costal cartilages of ribs seven through ten join together to insert at the inferior end of the sternal body.

Costochondral Joints

The articulations of the ribs and costal cartilages are the costochondral joints. They are synchondroses, without a synovial joint capsule. The costochondral joints can easily be disjointed by a sharp blow to the thorax. If you walk your fingers with some pressure along the surface of a rib, starting from the sternum, you can usually identify the point where the costal cartilage becomes bone. Depending upon your conformation, there will be a small indentation, ridge, or irregularity that marks the transition.

Sternocostal Joints

Between the sternum and the costal cartilages are the sternocostal joints. At the first rib, the joint is a synchondrosis and relatively immobile. From ribs two through seven, the joints are synovial. Aging affects the mobility of the sternocostal joints, and it is possible that the variations occur based on patterns of use, rendering a synovial joint cartilaginous if it does not move consistently.

Compression and Release: Ribs and Sternum

You can do this on yourself, but it can be rewarding to give and receive this touch with a partner. Locate the joint between your sternum and second rib at the sternal angle. Let the fingers of one hand be on your sternal angle and the other on the second rib, pointing toward each other. Slowly compress the joint space. Wait for a filling sensation to emerge and allow the joint to release, following the expansion with your fingers. Imagine that water, light, or air is filling the joint space. Notice the response in your body.

Moving down the sternum, repeat the compression and release at each sternocostal joint of that side. Notice the sensation of breath and movement on that side compared to the other, and then repeat on the second side.

Interchondral Joints

Joints that form between costal cartilages are called interchondral joints. The costal cartilage of the tenth rib joins with the costal cartilage of the ninth rib. That union joins with the eighth costal cartilage, and then with the seventh to insert on the sternum. There is an additional articulation between the sixth and seventh costal cartilages. Each of those articulations has a synovial joint that may become fibrous with lack of use or aging.

Moving the Ribs in the Planes

Enjoy differentiating your ribs from each other, and moving each one through all the planes. Try doing each of the following movements first with all the ribs of one side as a group, then differentiating lower, middle, and upper ribs, and final with focusing on each rib individually:

Vertical plane: lateral tilting.

Sagittal plane: flexion and extension of the trunk.

Horizontal plane: rotation.

Try the movements in varying relationships to the earth: standing, lying down on your back and then on your front, and on all fours.

Shining the Dome

With your partner sitting, place your hands on the lower ribs of one side of the ribcage. Map the upwardly tapering dome as it narrows under the armpits and shoulder girdle, imagining that you are shining the surface of the dome as you work. With your free hand lift your partner's shoulder to loosen the space under the shoulder girdle. With the active hand shine as many contours of the upper ribs as possible, to provide your partner's nervous system with sensory mapping of the dome. People have great sensitivity in this area, so proceed slowly. When you complete the first side do the same on the other, noticing together any differences between the sides. When finished, invite your partner to feel into the places where they were touched—the ribs—and allow the shoulder girdle to settle on them and find rest. Let the arms hang freely from the support of the dome.

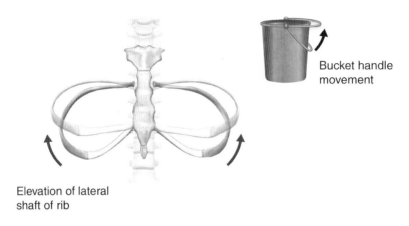

Elevation of lateral
shaft of rib

Bucket handle
movement

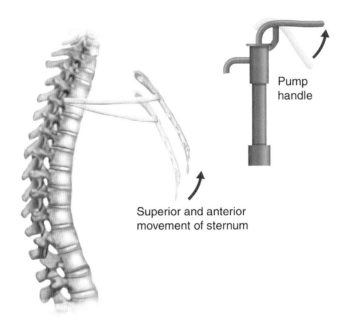

Superior and anterior
movement of sternum

Pump
handle

Figure 6.19

Rib motion

Breathing and the Ribs

The combined motion of costovertebral and costo-transverse articulations is rotation on the longitudinal axis of the rib's neck (Figure 6.18). The lower and middle ribs are designed to translate the rotation into a widening of the ribcage: expanding with in-breath to the sides and relaxing toward midline

on the exhalation. That motion is called the bucket handle image: the rib is attached front and back and opens to the side at its center point, tethered to its two attachments like a bucket handle being raised and lowered (Figure 6.19).

In the upper ribs, the motion of rotation at the articulation translates into a deepening of the upper thorax, which expands front to back with inhalation and condenses with exhalation. That sagittal plane motion is amplified by the sternal angle and the upper thoracic intervertebral joints, and is similar to the motion of a pump handle.

QR Code #7: Embodying the Bones of Breath

Bucket Handle Breathing

Balance the three curves of your spine while standing, sitting, or lying down. Envision your lower and middle ribs as handles of a bucket, with fixed points at the spine and at the sternum. Place the back of each hand on the corresponding side of your lower and middle ribs. Keeping the bucket handles in mind initiate the movement of in-breath by allowing your ribs to open and release to the sides. Then return to resting on the exhalation. This is especially freeing if the body has chosen a pattern of breathing that minimizes the motion of the ribs in the vertical plane.

Breathing in the Planes

One traditional approach to breathing is to fill the chest sequentially from the lower to middle to upper lungs and, in exhaling, to reverse that pattern, like a wave rolling up the beach and then retreating. You can enhance the pattern by differentiating the spatial contributions of your lower, middle, and upper ribs. The floating ribs expand in the horizontal plane as part of abdominal breathing. The tenth through fifth ribs participate in the vertical plane, while the upper four ribs ribs expand the chest sagitally.

Rising and Falling Breath

Take time to feel each component individually and then sequence the movement into a single breath: inhale and exhale. Enjoy!

Floating Ribs (The Horizontal Plane)

The inhalation in this breath can start with belly-breathing, if your belly is understood to include the entire circumference of the middle torso, not just the forward thrust of the abdomen. Allow your floating ribs to open like the page of a book from its spine, increasing the space in the back of your body as your belly moves forward and your sides open; this increases the capacity of the lower lobes of your lungs.

The Bucket Handle (The Vertical Plane)

After opening the space around the floating ribs, invite your breath to rise higher. Allow the lower and middle ribs to swing into width like a bucket handle and then release. This increases the capacity of the middle lobes of the lungs.

The Sternal Angle (The Sagittal Plane)

Finally allow your breath to rise as high as it can into the upper lungs and ribs. Enjoy the forward motion of your sternal body at the sternal angle as you inhale. Deepen the space between the front and back of your chest. On the exhalation, allow the bone to soften back to a resting position. This increases the capacity of the upper lobes of your lungs.

Global Breath

Global breathing is a simple, innocent breath, uninfluenced by our habits, traumas, histories, and intentions. It is the breath pattern of a healthy infant who experiences breath as a totality. In a global breath all of the support structures for the lungs initiate breath together, without a leader or a follower or a specific pattern, as in belly-breathing. All the ribs, the sternum, and the spine move simultaneously at each joint for the in-breath, as if a balloon were being blown up from its center point. The out-breath is a soft releasing of that global expansion, simultaneous in all our structures, with no pushing or forcing out of air (Douglas, 2004).

Exploring Global Breath

Make yourself comfortable in any position. Imagine that your thorax and abdomen form a nicely balanced round balloon. Inhaling into a center point of the sphere, deep to your xiphoid process, allow every surface of your thorax and abdomen to participate in a simultaneous expansion. Your entire front moves forward, your back (including the lumbar area) moves to the back, your sides move in their respective directions, and your shoulders release upward. Notice your habits of initiation compared to this global initiation. Notice your habits of release and where in your body you tend to hold, sustain, or pause during exhalation.

Extend the global pattern of your breath into your pelvis, including the pelvic floor, relaxing heel-wards during inhalation and coming to rest as you exhale.

Enjoying the Thorax

Bringing your awareness to your sternum, ribs, and thoracic spine, invite the bones and joints to initiate movement. Working with one bone or joint or many, invite the movement to sequence from the thorax into the entire body. Allow the bones to follow their own pleasure and logic in movement, releasing cognitive control for a while. What happens? Do you move in space or stay in place? Do you change levels, rising or falling, or stay at one level? Is the movement fast, slow, or something else? What patterns of movement emerge which surprise you? Which joints feel free, and which feel more restricted? How can breathing be a part of such movement? Can breathing initiate your movement?

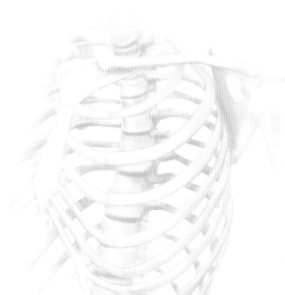

Integration: Hand to Ribs

Where the hands go, the eyes will follow
Where the eyes go, the mind will follow
Where the mind goes, emotions are evoked
Where the emotions move, the essence arises

yato hastas tato dṛiṣṭir
yato dṛiṣṭis tato manaḥ
yato manas tato bhāvo
yato bhāvas tato rasaḥ

– Nandikeshvara, 2nd century AD

The upper limbs are important actors in the cycle of being—the continuous process of sensing the environment, perceptual processing of that information, and moving in response to our interpretations of those stimuli. They allow us to protect and defend ourselves, to embrace each other and express our love, to work in the garden, to write, to change the world around us, to feed ourselves, and to fight when necessary. The movement habits of your upper extremities express your intention, state of mind, and relationship to the environment.

The bones and joints of the shoulder girdle and arms give each hand the remarkable ability to telescope smoothly away from the torso in a straight line in almost any direction in space. Each joint proximal to the carpal bones performs a role in the placement of the hand in space and contributes to its spatial intention: the ribs and shoulder girdle serve as a dynamic base of support for the shoulder joint; the elbow allows the hand to advance into space or retreat toward the body; and the forearm and wrist adjust the angle of the hand's approach.

Pleasure and Ease

Lie on your left side with your hips and knees bent. Let your left arm extend palm up at a 90 degree angle from your torso and support your head with a pillow if needed for comfort. Rest your right hand directly on top of your left, with elongated fingers. Keeping your right elbow elongated but not stiff, rotate your spine and shoulders so that the skin of your right hand slides back and forth against the skin of your left. Repeat as many times as you want. Enjoy the caress of your right hand on the skin of your left hand and arm. Let your right hand reach forward into space beyond the left hand and then retreat, sliding along the left wrist and forearm. Enjoy your breathing. Feel how the movement of your right hand creates movement in your shoulder girdle, chest, and spine. Maintaining the same movement, shift the point of initiation from your fingers to the space inside your chest cavity. Allow your arm, shoulder, and chest to relax and feel their weight.

When the sliding motion feels integrated and enjoyable, reach the fingers of your right hand forward in space one more time and then let them rise toward the ceiling, elevating your right arm. With the fingers flowing toward the ceiling, balance the sensation of the front of your shoulder with the sensation of the back of your shoulder. Then allow your fingers to retrace their pathway to the floor and slide again against the left hand. Repeat this rising and falling of your arm as many times as you like. Enjoy the sensations and invite your breath to support the movement.

When that motion feels integrated, allow your fingers to continue past the vertical and move behind your chest, maintaining the arm at shoulder level. Move your fingers as far behind you as you can comfortably. Allow the weight of the arm to open the shoulder girdle and ribs. Your right hand may or may not rest on the floor, but do not yet rotate your head. Use your breath to open the internal spaces of your chest and to relax any stretch that you may feel in your arm. Imagine wind between your joints, to give them more space. Initiating with a slight reach beyond your fingers, bring your arm back toward the ceiling and finally toward the floor, sliding once again across the left hand. Repeat as many times as you wish and finally let your head release with the hand.

When the opening of your hand and chest feels enjoyable and easy, add the focus of your eyes, which can travel with the fingers of your right hand in their wide arc up and across your chest. Notice how this changes the

experience. Allow your right hand to rest on the floor. Repeat as many times as you wish.

Finally, releasing the weight of your right arm against the floor, slowly slide your arm toward your head. (You might prefer to do that either in one smooth movement or in increments.) Allow your chest to move in response to the movement of your arm as your hand glides along the floor past your head and back to your left hand. Continue to use your breath as a support, and enjoy the gentle stretch and the weight of the movement.

Stand up and compare the sensation in your right arm and shoulder girdle with that in your left before you repeat on the other side.

Articular Pathway: Fingers to Spine

The numerous articulations between the tip of your finger and the spine provide flexibility and the possibility for the hand to move almost anywhere in space. The pathway is fairly direct from your distal phalanges to the carpus, wrist, elbow, and shoulder joint, but much less so from the shoulder to the spine. From the scapula, the pathway moves through the clavicle into the sternum, then to the ribs at the sternocostal joints, through the ribs to the back of the body and finally articulates with the spine. You can further specify the scapular contribution by mapping the route from the glenoid fossa down the lateral border to its tip, up the medial border to the spine of the scapula, across the spine to the acromion, and across the acromion to finally articulate with the clavicle at the acromioclavicular joint. Mary Lou Seereiter devised a wonderful way to use the sensory feedback of a small resilient ball against a wall to highlight the skeletal pathway between hand and spine. The following exploration is based on notes from one of her classes.

Fingers to Spine: Mary Lou's Ball Tracing

Beginning with your back against a wall and one arm at shoulder level, place a ball on the dorsum of your fingers. Move your body laterally so that the ball rolls across the back of your hand, forearm, and upper arm: feel the ball pressing into your bones. Arriving at your shoulder, shift your back upwards against the wall so that the ball traces the lateral border of your scapula down to the inferior angle. Continue shifting your body so that the pressure of the ball moves up the medial border to find the spine of the scapula, and shift across the scapular spine to the acromion. Now the tricky part: rotate your body carefully away from the wall but maintain contact with the ball so that it rolls across your acromion and acromioclavicular joint onto the clavicle. Your front surface will now be in contact with the wall. Pressing your weight into the ball, continue shifting so that it rides across your clavicle and sternoclavicular joint onto the sternum. Shift your body up along the wall so that the ball rolls down your sternum to the sixth or seventh rib. Rotating your body outward, enjoy the pressure as the ball traces the pathway of the rib around the side and back of your body: your arm will have to slide up the wall to accommodate the movement. As you face away from the wall with the ball approaching your spine, take a moment to visualize and feel the entire pathway from finger to spine. Repeat, improvise, enjoy, and notice any new sensations in your upper extremity before you do the other side.

Fingers to Spine: Mapping With a Partner

With a partner standing or sitting, map the bones along the pathway from fingers to spine. Wherever possible, invite movement at the joints through their full range of motion. You may wish to enhance the mapping with compression and expansion at some or all of the joints.

Moving Fingers to Spine

Hands Stabilized

Place your hands against a wall, the floor, or a partner, feeling the skeletal pathway from hands to spine. Maintain the fixed connection as you explore the many ways in which you can move your wrists, elbows, shoulder joints and girdle, ribs, and spine with stabilized hands. How does this feel? What does it make you want to do? Which joints and bones are the most active, and which bones and joints are less active?

Hands Free

Standing or walking, move your hands, arms, shoulders, and ribs through their full range of motion, aware of snaking pathway from fingers to spine. Reach for objects and release them, reach for others, and enjoy the power and mobility of your upper extremities. How does this feel? What does it make you want to do? Which joints and bones are the most active, and which bones and joints are less active?

Embodying Lines of Connection from the Fingers to the Scapula

As Martha Eddy outlines in her Foreword to this book, the felt-sense relationship between the scapula and hand and the lines of connection between specific areas of the scapula and individual fingers first originated with Irmgard Bartenieff and were then refined and elaborated by Bonnie Bainbridge Cohen. Based on my own experience and that of my students, exploring these skeletal relationships in movement is one of the most direct and pleasurable ways to embody the arms. The line of connection for mobility spirals from the radial hand and lateral arm to the anterior and superior shoulder girdle. The line of connection for stability spirals from the fourth and fifth fingers to the posterior and inferior portions of the scapula. The third finger plays a balancing role, mediating between the radial and ulnar hand. By enlivening those relationships the hand, arm, and scapula are able to function more efficiently. In your own research, you may feel different relationships between the hand and scapula but as a starting point for your inquiry, explore the ones below.

Table 7.1: Lines of Connection from Fingers to Shoulder Girdle

Finger	Forearm	Shoulder Girdle
Thumb	Radius	Coracoid process
Second finger	Radius	The V made by the scapular spine and clavicle
Third finger	The space between the radius and ulna	Glenoid fossa
Fourth finger	Ulna	Axillary border of the scapula
Fifth finger	Ulna	Inferior angle of the scapula

Embodying Lines of Connection: Fingers to Shoulder Girdle (Table 7.1)

Thumb

Bring your thumb to your coracoid process. Allow movement to emerge as they touch. Gradually let the thumb move away from the coracoid process, maintaining a flow of energy between them. Ask the thumb to lead the arm into space. What gestures emerge? How does the thumb want to express itself? What parts of your torso become involved? Does the movement emphasize space toward the front of the body, toward the back of the body, or something in-between?

Index Finger

Begin by feeling how the spine of the scapula and the clavicle form a V, pointing toward the hand. Continue that line of energy through arm into the index finger and sense the pointing of the index finger as though it emerges directly out of the V of the shoulder girdle. Allow movement to connect the finger and the V. What gestures emerge? How does the finger want to express itself? How do you use the space around you most easily—near the body, in a middle range, or far from the body?

Middle Finger

Begin by sensing a line of flow from the center of the glenoid fossa through the space between the ulna and radius, into the capitate bone, and the middle finger. Maintaining this connection, allow the finger to initiate movement in space and as an axis for rotation of the forearm. Do the hand and shoulder joint feel balanced? What kind of movement and gesture emerge from this connection? How does it change the way you use space around you?

Fourth Finger

Begin by sensing a flow of connection from the lateral border of the scapula through the humerus into the ulna and the fourth finger. As the finger moves, sense the diagonal of the axillary border supporting freedom of movement into space. How does that movement differ from movement initiated from the third finger? Is it freer spatially? Pterosaurs (flying dinosaurs) flew from wings attached to the fourth digit. Does the lightness of flight emerge from your fourth finger-to-scapula connection?

Little Finger

Begin by connecting the inferior angle of your scapula through the humerus into the ulna and little finger. Maintain that sensation as you alternate drawing the little finger closer to you and pressing it away from your body. Begin to explore the space around you, and see what movement emerges as you maintain the connection. Allow your hand to support your weight on the floor, and feel the relationship between the inferior angle of the scapula and the little finger. Is it more constrained than the movement from the ring finger? What gestures or patterns of movement emerge? How does the finger want to express itself? How do you use the space around you?

Charting Lines of Connection from Fingers to Shoulder Girdle

With your partner standing, sitting, or side lying on the floor, use your fingers or a brush to lightly chart the connection pathway from each finger to the scapula. Find a route that makes sense to you and your partner. Try tracing the pathway on the back of the arm as well as on the front. Adjust to your partner's appetite for touch: deeper, lighter, faster, or slower. Explore and enjoy the following suggestions:

- Use different qualities of touch to bring awareness to the connections

- Map the bones in both directions, from finger to scapula and scapula to finger

- Invite your partner to move the arm and shoulder girdle in response to your touch

- Have a group of small objects available for your partner to pick up and handle, using the sensory connections you are working on

- Complete all the pathways of one arm, and invite your partner to notice how that arm feels in comparison to the untreated arm.

Embodying Lines of Connection from Fingers to Ribs

At birth, an infant's fingers tend to be closed around its palm, and the hand functions as a unit. From the tight palmar grasp, the little finger opens first and the fingers open sequentially toward the thumb, which is the last digit to become active. While the hand is developing in that sequence, an infant is simultaneously developing the strength to lift its head away from the earth and eventually to use its hands and arms to push the upper body away from the earth. The process requires control of the ribs, starting from the uppermost rib downward. The simultaneous development of the fingers and ribs are mutually supportive. As adults, we benefit from reestablishing the parallel individuation of the fingers and the ribs (Bainbridge Cohen, 1995, p. 31).

The function of the ulnar hand relates to the function of ribs one through four. The function of the radial hand relates to the use of the lower ribs, five through twelve. The specific relationships between the individual fingers and ribs are shown in Table 7.2.

Table 7.2: Lines of Connection from Fingers to Ribs

Finger	Ribs
Fifth finger	Ribs 1 and 2
Fourth finger	Ribs 3 and 4
Third finger	Ribs 5 and 6
Second finger	Ribs 7 to 10
Thumb	Ribs 11 and 12

Lines of Connection: Pushing from the Floor

Lying prone, with palms down and head to one side, take time to sink into relationship with the floor. Relax your belly and spread your fingers.

Press gently against the floor with your fifth finger. Allow the activation to change the tone of your arms, tracking activation through your arms to your first and second ribs. Create just enough pressure to lift up your first and second ribs and shift your head from one side to the other, like a newborn baby—your nose will just miss the floor.

Add downward pressure in your fourth finger, finding a line of connection into the third and fourth ribs. Allow your chest to rise a little higher as you turn it, but not so much that the movement goes into lower ribs.

Add pressure in the third finger, activating the fifth and sixth ribs. Rise even higher without disturbing the ribs below.

Add pressure in the index finger, activating the seventh through tenth ribs: you will be able to move to the bottom of your sternum and area beneath your scapula. Your head will move higher still.

Finally, add pressure in the thumb, inviting the activation to flow into your floating ribs, and rise a little higher in space. Using the whole hand and all of your ribs, your eyes will likely be at the horizontal, enabling you to scan the room.

The Axial Skeleton and Skull

The spine, the spinal column, the backbone, the vertebral column—all are terms for the bony axis that provides our central organization. Humans alone have spines and skulls fully adapted to the habit of upright gait: we are the only species to experience life primarily on the vertical. The achievement of walking with an upright spine is a developmental landmark in each human's life, involving complex neurological coordination of reflexes, righting reactions, movement constellations, and muscular control. Such locomotion elevates the head with its special senses and frees the hands, offering a completely flexible relationship with the environment.

Embodying the Vertebral Column

The 33 segments of the vertebral column are amazingly mobile when they are balanced and free to articulate. What we call a straight spine is actually a delicately counterbalanced series of curves, supporting a structural matrix of fascia and soft tissues that extends well beyond the physical boundaries of the vertebrae. The discs that separate the segments provide cushioning and add resilience to the structure. When we bring awareness to these elements of the central axis, profound changes can occur, affecting the efficiency of breathing, ease of movement, and the health of the entire body.

Each vertebral segment is unique in its morphology, its proportions, and its role in the spinal column. Vertebral segments belonging to each region—cervical, thoracic, and lumbar—share characteristics that distinguish them from segments belonging to the other regions. Nevertheless, there are elements that are common to almost all the vertebrae (Figure 8.1). Those features include:

- A vertebral body that provides the stability of weight bearing: it participates with other segments in the longitudinal column of support. The higher in the spinal column, the smaller and more delicate the vertebral body is. The lowest segments of the lumbar spine are quite massive relative to the uppermost.

- A vertebral foramen, the round space for the passage of the spinal cord.

- A vertebral arch forming a ring around the vertebral foramen.

- Pedicles that extend symmetrically from the vertebral body to the transverse processes.

- Laminae that extend posteriorly from the transverse processes to meet in the back and close the arch.

- Superior and inferior articular processes extending from the junction of each pedicle and lamina. The superior processes rise to present a surface (an articular facet) that articulates with the vertebral segment above, and the inferior processes descend to bear a surface that articulates with the vertebral segment below.

- Superior and inferior articular facets on the articular processes, forming the points of contact with neighboring bones.

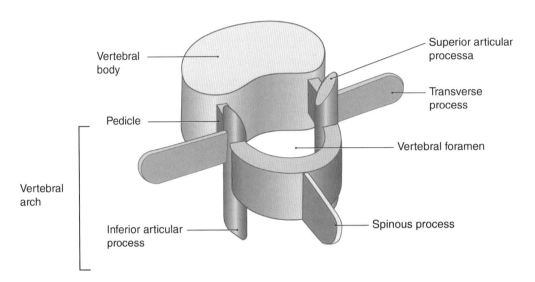

Figure 8.1

Generalized vertebra

- Transverse processes, projecting laterally from the junction of the pedicle and lamina and serving as muscle attachments.

- A spinous process projecting dorsally from the junction of the two laminae. The part of the spine that is easily palpable, it serves as a site for muscle attachments.

As a whole, the vertebral column is capable of moving in flexion and extension, side bending (lateral flexion), and rotation—and in complex combinations of those movements. The facet joints between vertebral segments allow for varying degrees of motion in each of those directions. If motion becomes limited by postural habits, inadequate organ support, or for other reasons, the spine can accommodate and stabilize in the shape of the habit. These habitual accommodations become problematic: scoliosis is a lateral curve in the spine, often with some degree of rotation in the affected segments; kyphosis is an excess flexion or rounding of the spine at any level; and lordosis is the habit of excess extension, usually seen in the lumbar spine.

Mobilizing the Vertebral Column

In supine, roll a small resilient ball the length of your spine, from coccyx to occiput. Release your weight into the ball at every level and bring awareness to your breath, pausing wherever you like to connect with yourself and the earth. Continue to use contact with the ball for mobility as you do the rest of the exploration.

Cervical Spine

Breathe into your soft palate and low brain. Begin moving in those areas, and use that small but luscious movement to enhance ease and mobility in your atlanto-occipital joint. Rest and breathe.

Then touch your hyoid bone while sensing and moving the back of your mouth (oropharynx and nasopharynx). Use this awareness to soften and mobilize your upper cervical spine, C1 to C3, taking time to explore whatever movement is available and to invite delicious articulation between the vertebrae. Then touch the point of your thyroid cartilage, sensing your laryngopharynx, and gently move the muscles of swallowing: use this awareness to mobilize the middle cervical spine, C3 to C5, opening to ease and fluidity. Move your hand lower to touch the front of your neck over your thyroid gland, softening your trachea and esophagus. Mobilize the facet joints from C5 to C7, enjoying the relaxation and mobility of all the cervical vertebrae and discs.

Thoracic Spine

Place your hand on the base of your neck, your clavicle and the manubrium of your sternum, feeling your thymus and the top of your lungs. Use the sensations to gently mobilize your upper thoracic spine, T1 to T4, taking your time to feel micro-movements and fluid irrigation of the area. Then move your hand down to your sternal body, encouraging your heart, lungs, aorta, and esophagus to move internally: use this motility to find flow in the joints and discs of your mid-thoracic spine, T5 to T8. Shift your hand once again just below your sternum, over your upper abdominal organs. Sliding your liver, stomach, pancreas, and upper intestines, feel your internal fluidity, and take this awareness further back to the anterior surface of your lower thoracic spine, T9 to T12. Allow the discs and joints of your entire thoracic spine to enjoy their mobility.

Lumbar Spine

Place your hand on your belly at your navel. Feel the relaxation and depth of your small intestines, your kidneys, and the pancreas. Let them fall against the upper part of your lumbar spine, L1 to L3, and use the sensation to find movement at the thoracolumbar junction between T12 and L1, and below. Feel the marshmallow texture of your discs and the fluidity of your intervertebral joints. Move your hands once again to the space between your navel and pubic bone. Use the touch to feel into the deeper digestive organs, the colon and lower small intestines. As you mobilize those deep organs enjoy the mobility of L3 to L5, the sliding of the facet joints, and open up the space at the lumbosacral joint between L5 and S1.

Take some time to indulge in movement, breath, and vibration of your spinal column as a whole. When finished, notice what feels different and how your movement in space has been affected.

Stability and Mobility

As we embody the spine, it is important to differentiate between the parts of it primarily meant for weight bearing and those that facilitate movement. The chunky block-like vertebral bodies are adapted to the work of transmitting weight into the earth and providing stability. The vertebral processes, delicate wing-like structures in the back of the spine, provide attachments for ligaments and muscles and are adapted to the function of mobility. Spinal dysfunction and much pain can arise out of confusion—in posture and movement—between spinal mobility and spinal stability.

QR Code #8: Embodying the Vertebral Column

For many people, the word back is synonymous with the spinal column, because when we touch the center of our backs, we encounter a bone. What we touch at the back is actually the spinous process, part of the mobility structure of the vertebral column. The vertebral bodies that form the weight-bearing column are actually closer to the center of the torso, not at the posterior surface. As a result, when we are instructed to stand up straight a common response is to throw our shoulders back, place our weight behind the vertebral bodies, and force the muscles and the more delicate parts of the vertebrae to act as weight-bearing bones. In yoga, dance, and martial arts instruction, we are sometimes encouraged to do just that. Unfortunately, that stance forces weight onto the structures behind the vertebral bodies meant for mobility. It requires muscular tension to sustain and compresses the space between vertebral segments, compensations that eventually lead to back pain and reduced mobility.

Standing Forward Roll Downs: Spinous Processes and Vertebral Bodies

Standing comfortably in a parallel position of the feet, touch and bring awareness to the spinous processes in the back of your body. Starting with your atlanto-occipital joint, allow your head to incline forward. Continue the motion sequentially through the cervical spine, initiating by opening the spaces between the spinous processes. Continue to work segment by segment through the thoracic spine: fold at your hips, knees, and ankles if you feel any strain in your back. Continue to work through your lumbar segments, and by this time you will be folded forward with your head dangling and arms releasing toward the floor.

Again, roll down your spine from standing, but this time locate your cervical vertebral bodies within yourself, right in the center of your neck. Initiating from there, allow your head to relax downward, moving this time from the front of your cervical spine, the surface that nestles against your esophagus. Sequence through each of your thoracic and lumbar vertebral bodies and notice the difference in sensation and quality of movement when you initiate from your vertebral bodies as compared to the spinous processes.

Curves of the Spine

Each region of the vertebral column is associated with a curve moving through the sagittal plane in such a way that alternating curves undulate along the length of the spine (Figure 8.2). The cervical curve is convex to the front, the thoracic curve is concave, the lumbar curve is convex, and the sacrum is again concave to the front. The concavity of the back of the skull counterbalances the concavity of the sacrum. Balancing the front and back of the body, these five curves are mutually supportive: if one curve is limited, strained, or displaced, other areas of the spine will be forced to compensate for the deviation.

Developmentally, we emerge from the womb with a single curve hollowing the front of the body, the primary curve. As newborns develop the ability to lift their heads from the ground, they accumulate the strength to sustain a cervical curve that helps to hold the head up. Later, as they push away from the earth, the lumbar curve emerges as a support for locomotion. The thoracic spine, sacrum, and back of the skull retain the shape of the primary curve throughout life. Occasionally, the stresses of aging return older adults toward the expression of the primary curve, where the back is rounded from head to tail.

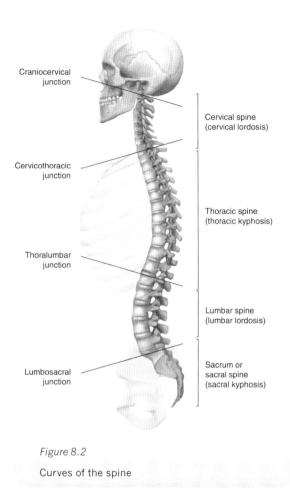

Craniocervical
junction

Cervical spine
(cervical lordosis)

Cervicothoracic
junction

Thoracic spine
(thoracic kyphosis)

Thoralumbar
junction

Lumbar spine
(lumbar lordosis)

Lumbosacral
junction

Sacrum or
sacral spine
(sacral kyphosis)

Figure 8.2

Curves of the spine

Establishing the Spinal Curves: Child's and Table Poses

Rest on the floor in child's pose, and enjoy breathing in the primary curve of the spine from head to tail. Bring awareness to sounds and smells, and allow your curiosity about what you sense around you to elevate your head slowly from the floor. As your head rises, feel the secondary curve becoming established in the cervical spine.

Carefully and slowly experiment with rising to table position on all fours, feeling the lumbar curve establish itself. Many people retain a flexed position in the lumbar spine, thinking that it is straight: check in a mirror or ask a friend to help you establish the lumbar curve if you have questions about it. In table position, feel the alternating curves: occipital, cervical, thoracic, lumbar, and sacral working together to support the trunk. Imagine that the sacrum, thorax, and occiput subtly retain child's pose while the cervical and lumbar spine create table position.

Establishing the Spinal Curves: Locomotion

When your curves are well established on all fours, experiment with cross-lateral creeping. If your curves are balanced, the movement can be easy and well coordinated. The movement will feel more awkward if you retain lumbar flexion, a collapsed thorax, or a distortion of your cervical curve.

Sit back on your heels and bring the balance of the three curves into a vertical relationship with gravity. Can you feel the curves balancing the front and back of your body, and can you feel the transition points between the various curves? Those points are the lumbosacral junction, where the sacrum and lumbar spine meet; the thoracolumbar junction, where the lumbar curve transitions into the thoracic; and the cervicothoracic junction at C7-T1, where the thoracic kyphosis transitions into the cervical lordosis.

Rise to standing and see if you can retain your sensitivity to the design and sensation of the curves.

Aligning the Spinal Curves on the Vertical

As we come to standing we have the challenge of meeting gravity through the curves of the spine. To find a structurally ideal alignment we might drop a plumb line from a point between the atlanto-occipital joints, where the skull meets the cervical spine. That line would then fall through the vertebral bodies of the neck, a bit anterior to the thoracic vertebral bodies, through the center of the lumbar segments, and down through the centered balance point of the ischial tuberosities. Sensing weight flow through those points can support effortless spinal alignment (Berland, 2017).

If the plumb line is in order, then each spinal curve will have a segment at its apex: the anterior surface of that vertebral body will face forward, parallel to the earth, while the other vertebral surfaces are at various angles depending upon the shape of your curves (Figure 8.3). You can determine in your own

body what those vertebrae might be, but generally L3 is the apex of the lumbar curve, T6 or T7 is the apex of the thoracic curve, and C4 is the apex of the cervical.

Neutral Spine

Stand in a comfortable position and feel your vertebral bodies. Become aware of your head balancing on the atlanto-occipital joints deep to your mastoid processes. Feel or imagine the weight of your head flowing through the center of your cervical bodies, just in front of your thoracic bodies (through the back of your heart), and through the center of your lumbar bodies, before flowing through your sitting bones and into your legs and feet. Can you sustain this feeling while walking, running, moving, or dancing?

Alternatively, identify the anterior surface of C4 (just at the level of the top of your thyroid cartilage); the anterior surface of T6 or T7 (at or near the level of the midpoint of your sternal body); and the anterior surface of L3 (deep to your navel). Sense simultaneously into those points, and experiment with them to refine the alignment of the curves of your spine.

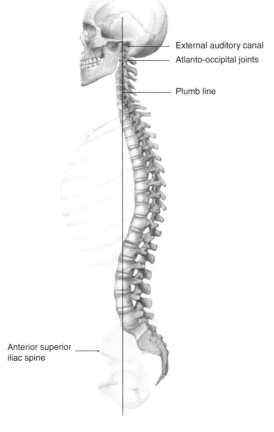

External auditory canal
Atlanto-occipital joints

Plumb line

Anterior superior
iliac spine

Figure 8.3

Spinal plumb line

Embodying the Cervical Vertebrae

The seven cervical vertebrae are the smallest and most delicate of the spinal segments. They are larger in the horizontal dimension than in the vertical or sagittal. Collectively, they form a pedestal for the skull and permit its movement. The first and second segments have specialized roles in relationship to the movement of the head, and are therefore shaped differently from the others. The seventh is also unique as a transitional segment, sharing some characteristics with the thoracic vertebrae.

The cervical transverse processes possess an anterior costal element (this becomes the rib in the

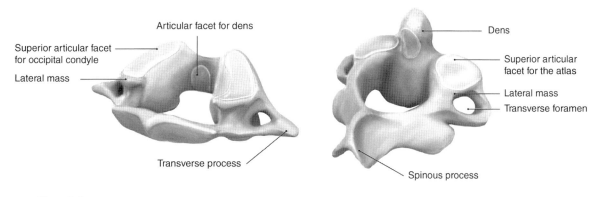

Figure 8.4

Atlas and axis

thoracic vertebrae), a posterior vertebral element, and between them the foramen transversarium, a passageway for autonomic nerves and the vertebral artery and vein. The spinous process in the cervical area is short, tapered, and often split into two portions at the end.

The Atlas

The first cervical vertebra (C1) is the atlas, named for its role in holding up the globe of the head (Figure 8.4). It resembles a ring with little wings. It lacks a vertebral body and a spinous process, instead having an anterior arch that, together with the posterior arch, encircles the vertebral foramen. Its paired superior and paired inferior articular facets are found on the lateral masses, which are widened areas between the anterior and posterior arches.

The superior articular facet is concave and receives the condyles of the occipital bone of the skull. The articulation with the occiput is called the atlanto-occipital joint. Its motion is through the sagittal plane, allowing the head to nod yes. Freedom of movement at the atlanto-occipital joint in both extension and flexion is important for the flow of fluids, nerves, and energy through the cranial base. It functions in reciprocity with the temporomandibular joint.

The inferior articular facet is nearly flat and circular. It forms part of the atlanto-axial joint with the second cervical vertebra, and is responsible for 50 percent of the rotary motion in the neck, allowing the head to indicate no. The articular surfaces are close to the horizontal, unlike the articular surfaces of subsequent vertebra, which are shaped to allow motion in all the planes.

The Axis

The second cervical vertebra (C2) is called the axis (Figure 8.4). From its body a tooth-like projection, the dens, extends vertically through the ring of the atlas toward the head. It provides a pivot point for the atlanto-axial joint's rotation and a third point of articulation between the atlas and the axis.

The Sixth Cervical Vertebra

The sixth cervical vertebra (C6) uniquely possesses symmetrical knob-like protrusions called the carotid tubercles, which extend laterally from the articular processes. They are palpable through the muscles from the front of the neck, at the level of the first cricoid ring under the thyroid cartilage.

Palpation and Location of the Cervical Vertebrae

The cervical vertebrae are located in the relatively slender neck and so are more available to touch than most. Palpate the following cervical structures in your own or a partner's body:

- The transverse processes of C1: find the mastoid process of the temporal bone, draw a line from there to the angle of the jaw, move your fingers halfway down that line, and press firmly to find the processes. You will be able to control rotation of the head by rotating the processes.

- The transverse processes of all the cervical vertebrae (as a ridge).

- The spinous processes from C2 through C7. Note that C7 has a significantly larger spinous process than the higher cervical vertebrae.

- Note that C3 is deep to the hyoid bone.

- Note that the intervertebral space between C4 and C5 is deep to the point of the thyroid cartilage.

- Note that the body of C6 is deep to the first cricoid ring. The carotid tubercle is found laterally at the same level.

Finding Yes and No

Yes!

The atlanto-occipital joint provides the rocking yes motion of the head (Figure 8.5). Identify the level of the joint by placing your fingers at the mastoid process on each side of your skull. Stabilize your cervical vertebrae by placing your hands on your neck, to inhibit movement. Gently find the gliding yes movement of the atlanto-occipital joint; see if any of the surrounding tissues relax.

No!

The atlanto-axial joint provides the pivoting no motion of the head. Stabilize the other cervical vertebrae by placing your hands on your neck. Gently find the gliding no movement of the atlanto-axial joint. Carefully alternate between yes and no, and invite the awareness that the movement of the atlanto-occipital joint occurs at a slightly higher level in the spine than the movement of the atlanto-axial joint.

Atlanto-Occipital Mobilization

With your partner lying supine, sit comfortably so that you can support the weight of the skull in both hands. Encourage the release of the head into your hands. With your index fingers, identify the deep crease at the base of the skull. Deep to that is the atlas. Then place your index fingers on

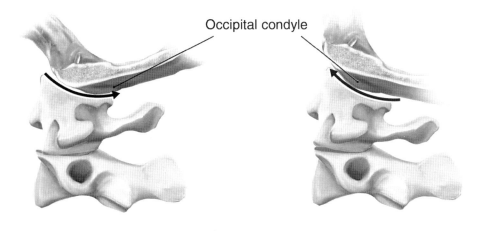

Occipital condyle

Flexion at the atlanto-occipital joint   Extension at the atlanto-occipital joint

Figure 8.5

Motion at the atlanto-occipital joint

the mastoid processes of the temporal bones, and ask your partner to imagine or feel the atlanto-occipital joints on the line between your fingers.

Having established the location of the atlanto-occipital joints, work with a very small motion at first, gliding the occipital condyles over the joint surfaces of the atlas, alternating slight flexion with slight extension. Remember that the motion is an arc, with the convex condyles of the occiput rotating in the concave receptacles of the atlas.

The AO joint will be free in some people and more limited in others. Ask your partner how the exploration feels, and how it affects the rest of their body. Invite them to perform the same small motions while sitting or standing.

Embodying the Thoracic Vertebrae

The 12 thoracic vertebrae form the longest portion of the spine as well as the posterior chest cavity. Each thoracic segment has a companion rib and with the sternum, the entire structure protects the heart, lungs, and other organs.

The thoracic spine retains the primary curve of the spine, creating a hollow within which the heart and lungs can nestle. A steep downward angle of the spinous processes limits extension, but allows for some degree of additional flexion. Rotation is permitted at all the intervertebral joints, and lateral flexion is relatively free.

The vertebral bodies increase in size from the relatively small T1 to the large T12. The second through ninth segments each have superior and inferior costal facets on each side of the body to articulate with the heads of the ribs. Each of those segments therefore contacts two ribs, one on the superior aspect and one on the inferior. The first, 11th, and 12th vertebrae articulate with only one rib.

Moving the Thoracic Spine

Touch T1 with one hand and T12 with the other. Maintaining your touch at those levels, enjoy rotation, flexion/extension, and lateral bending of the thoracic spine, while limiting movement in your cervical and lumbar regions. Notice your breath as you initiate from the vertebral bodies, and again as you initiate from your spinous processes.

Move into flexion by allowing the thoracic spine to fold around your heart, and move into extension by releasing the heart from your spine's embrace. Then initiate from your heart: move it backward into the spine and feel the vertebrae soften and fold in response. Find thoracic extension by allowing your heart to move forward in space: let the spinal segments respond.

Like all the vertebrae, each thoracic segment has a pedicle and a lamina on each side, forming the vertebral arch that surrounds the vertebral foramen. At the junction of the pedicle and lamina are three projections: the transverse process and the superior and inferior articular processes. The thoracic transverse processes project on a diagonal, both laterally and posteriorly. They are quite prominent, except at T11 and T12, where they are diminished in size.

Transverse Processes: Side Bending

Imagine that your thoracic spine is a telephone pole, and that your transverse processes are the spikes in its side that allow linemen to climb the pole. Initiate side bending by moving the spikes on one side of the pole away from each other and condensing the opposite spikes toward each other. Maintain awareness of all the spikes, and feel the malleability of the pole. Return to the vertical by reversing the process. What is the sensation of side bending from your transverse processes? How is it different from your normal movement?

Repeat the process, and add the transverse processes of your cervical and lumbar vertebral segments.

The spinous processes from T1 through T10 descend from their vertebral bodies like tails; the tip of each process is at the same level as the body of the vertebral segment below it. T11 and T12 are transitional to lumbar conformation, having spinous processes that project posteriorly rather than inferiorly. In all the thoracic vertebrae, the posterior surface of the process is ridged, tapering from a broad superior portion to a narrowed inferior tip.

The twelfth thoracic vertebra plays an important role in integration of the upper and lower body. At that point muscles that support and move the arms and legs meet—the upper portion of the iliopsoas muscle and the lower portion of the latissimus dorsi muscle—and it offers a posterior attachment for the breathing diaphragm.

Embodying the Lumbar Vertebrae

The bodies of the five lumbar vertebrae are massive, with relatively short processes posterior to the vertebral foramen. These are the large building blocks of the spinal column, supporting a much greater accumulated weight from higher in the body than do the cervical or thoracic vertebrae. The vertebral foramen is smaller in proportion to the size of the vertebra in the lumbar segments than in the cervical or thoracic segments. The pedicles of the lumbar vertebral arches are short and thick. The laminae are short and form a broad plate, merging with the spinous process.

The lateral processes that emerge from the lumbar vertebral arches are called costal processes, because they derive from ribs that have fused with the arch. The actual transverse processes are vestigial, projecting from the side of the superior articular process. The superior and inferior articular processes resemble those in the thoracic vertebrae, but the articular facets are rounded (the superior facets are concave and the inferior are convex) and no longer close to the vertical plane. The spinous processes are short and project dorsally.

Some degree of movement is available in each plane. Flexion is limited, but the articular facets permit a great deal of extension. The curved shape of the articular facets permits both rotation and a small amount of lateral flexion.

Moving the Lumbar Spine

Touch L1 with one hand and L5 with the other. Enjoy rotation, flexion/extension, and lateral bending of the lumbar spine while limiting thoracic and cervical movement. Then allow the movement of your lumbar spine to sequence throughout the column and into your limbs. What happens to your pelvis? To your hips and legs? How does the lumbar spine move while you walk?

In table position, initiate cat and cow movement (flexion and extension) by moving the lumbar spine and allowing it to ripple through your body.

In supine, notice the curve of your lumbar spine. Increase it and feel how it affects your neck and thorax. Decrease it and notice the difference. Balance the center of the sacrum on the floor and notice how your lumbar curve feels.

Tail Wagging

Sitting on a physioball, allow your sitting bones to release down toward the earth and your head to rise easily from your spine. Begin moving the coccyx, your tail, slightly forward and backward. Gradually increase the movement so that your lumbar spine is rocking as well, inhibiting motion in your shoulders and upper torso. Then wag your tail side to side, enjoying lateral movement in the lumbar spine. Combine those movements to create circles and figure eights, maintaining initiation from your coccyx.

The Intervertebral Discs

Some of our sea-dwelling ancestors had resilient stiffening rods called notochords separating the digestive system in the front of the body from the central nervous system in the back of the body (Dimon, 2011, pp. 25–30). In more highly developed fish, and eventually in the creatures that emerged from the sea onto land, bony vertebral segments further strengthened the rod, and together formed a vertebral column as a foundation for more complex movement and for resisting the pull of gravity. The remnants of the notochord are still found within us as the nucleus pulposus, the central part of the intervertebral disc that provides cushioning, resilience, and juiciness for spinal movement (Figure 8.6).

The discs are composed of a tough outer layer, the annulus fibrosis, and a gelatinous core, the nucleus pulposus. Each disc, interposed between two vertebral segments, has two vertebral attachments, one inferior and one superior. The front and back surfaces of each disc are also attached to the longitudinal ligaments of the spine. They are like elastic cushions that function as shock absorbers and make up about 25 percent of the length of the spinal column. Imagine a marshmallow sitting between each of your vertebral bodies: it responds to the movement of the spine by compressing and then rebounding to its original shape upon release.

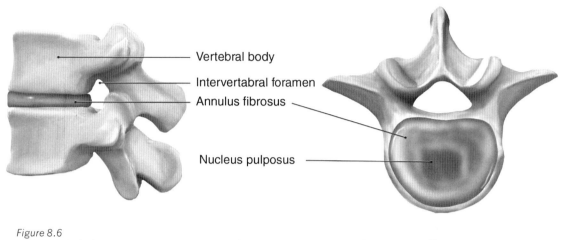

Vertebral body

Intervertabral foramen

Annulus fibrosus

Nucleus pulposus

Figure 8.6

Intervertebral disc

The juicy, buoyant quality of the discs can be lost with age, as the nucleus pulposus shrinks or dries out, leading to a process of ossification of parts of the disc. Healthy discs shrink less with aging!

Movement of the spine in any direction requires the discs to accommodate the changing spaces between the vertebrae. It is important to keep the weight centered through the vertebral bodies, so that the discs do not become habitually compressed on one side so that they displace and interfere with the spinal cord or adjacent nerve roots. Maintaining equilibrium in the discs keeps the spine resilient and juicy.

Weight Flow Through the Discs

Stand behind your partner and place your hands symmetrically on their shoulders, close to the neck. Gradually increase your downward pressure, directing it through your partner's vertebral bodies and discs. If your partner feels extra pressure or compression in the small of the back, the sacrum, or the heels, the weight is not flowing through the discs. Release the pressure and invite your partner to reposition their weight a little forward so that the force moves through the discs. When the pressure flows through the discs, your touch will connect through the legs and spread through the feet into the floor without forcing pressure into the back surface of the body. Bring awareness to the marshmallows!

The Integrated Spine

You can embody your spine at the level of a single vertebra and its parts, at the level of a region of the spine, or as an integrated whole. As previously noted, spinal embodiment and alignment facilitates movement of the entire body. The following explorations offer approaches to working with the column as a functional unit.

Moving from Sacrum and Occiput

Place one hand on your occiput and one hand on your sacrum. Sense the solidity of the vertebral bodies and the fluidity of the intervertebral discs. Move your entire spine through all the planes, initiating equally from the sacrum and from the occiput. Enjoy the movement.

Touching Sacrum and Occiput

With your partner supine, place one hand under the sacrum and the other beneath the occiput. Maintain that position, feeling your partner's breath and allowing for a flow of energy and relationship between those two points. Notice any subtle movement that occurs in bones or torso.

Seated Weight Flow Through the Spine

Sit comfortably on a chair with a relatively hard surface but do not use the backrest. Rest your feet on the floor. Sense the curves of your spine. Rock your pelvis slightly by rolling over the curved surface of the ischial tuberosities, allowing them to drop into the earth through the chair. Finally come to a balanced position of the pelvis on the sitting bones, with the pelvis neither tucked back in posterior pelvic tilt nor tilted forward in anterior pelvic tilt.

Allow your weight to pour into your pelvis through the vertebral bodies (closer to the center of the torso), being careful that the weight is not being dropped through the spinous processes or through the vertebral foramina. Acknowledge each curve in the spine.

At each vertebral level, balance the sensation in the front of your body with the sensation in the back of your body, feeling the vertebral bodies as a central support.

Facilitating Seated Weight Flow Through the Spine

Invite your partner to sit comfortably on a chair with a relatively hard surface, with feet fully on the floor. Prepare the spine by asking your partner to rock slightly over the sitting bones, allowing them to drop into the earth through the chair. Make sure that the pelvis is resting on the sitting bones, neither tucked back nor tilted forward, and that the three curves of the spine are balanced. Help your partner to feel the vertebral bodies (rather than the spinous processes) carrying the weight through the trunk into the sacrum and pelvis.

With an extremely light touch, place one hand on the front of your partner's upper chest and the other on the back at the same level. Ask whether your partner feels your anterior or posterior hand more, or whether the sensation coming from your two hands is the same? If there is an imbalance, ask your partner to shift slightly in space, or to bring more awareness to the surface through the breath. When sensation is diminished in the back, people will often move in that direction. You might suggest a forward repositioning instead, to see if the vertebral column will take the weight and allow the back to release into sensation.

Repeat, moving down the spine, balancing awareness of front and back in order to facilitate the movement of weight through the vertebral bodies.

Return to the upper chest, and repeat the process, moving up the cervical spine. Finish by balancing the front and back of the head.

Spinal Tap

Position your partner in side lying, comfortably supported with pillows under the head and between the knees. Identify and touch the spinous process of T1. Visualize the slight upward diagonal from the spinous process to the body, moving your energy along the diagonal and imagining that the bone is softening. Then with your thumb or a pair of fingers add some pressure, directing it gently but deeply toward the vertebral body. Feel the pressure penetrating the vertebral body, and sense a small forward displacement of the individual segment in response to your touch. Notice whether there is a rebound when you release your pressure and whether the segment feels individuated.

Repeat with each thoracic and lumbar vertebra, moving tailward. Remember that pressure on the spinous process of a thoracic vertebral segment will result in movement at a higher level, because of the downward sweep of the spinous tail. Adjust your touch to reflect that, so that the pressure moves upward on a diagonal to reach the vertebral body. In the lumbar vertebrae, the spinous processes extend dorsally from the vertebral bodies, so the pressure can be directed anteriorly.

Take it slowly, and notice if the vertebral segment you are working with is willing to move or is immobile, and whether there is ease or a sense of soreness or discomfort in your partner's back at this level. Invite your partner to move when finished, and to notice any changes in the sensation of movement.

Embodying the Skull

The 22 bones of the human skull perform a wide variety of functions. They are arranged in an incredibly complex spatial design, with numerous and intricate joints, and intimate relationships with all the other systems of the body. A portion of the skull is dedicated to protecting the nervous system. Another portion participates in the digestive system by providing its entry point and chewing mechanism, and the respiratory system by providing the breathing passageway. The skull is also the skeletal foundation for the senses of sight, smell, taste, hearing, and proprioception. Like the bones of the hands, the skull allows us to grasp and release with the jaw. Like the bones of the feet, the skull allows us to stand, as long as we are agile enough to balance on our heads. Those functions and many more are performed by two groups of bones: the facial bones, those supporting the digestive and respiratory functions; and the cranial bones, those primarily supporting and protecting the brain (Figure 8.7).

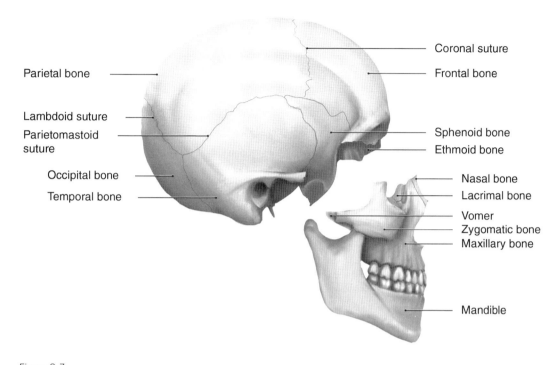

Figure 8.7

Cranial and facial bones

Mapping Cranial and Facial Bones

Touching gently, map the small, delicate, intricately shaped bones underneath your eyes and around your nose, mouth, and jaw. Notice the complexity of their design and the many surfaces available to touch. Move the bones in space. How does it feel to awaken their self-awareness?

Then with a light touch map the large bones protecting your brain. Feel the contours of the surface of the cranium on the front, top, sides, and back of your head. Move the bones in space. How does it feel to enliven the cranial bones? Can you separate the cranium from the facial bones in your sensory map of yourself? Enjoy the feeling of bringing awareness to different parts of the skull, sensing how the bones support your thinking, breathing, seeing, hearing, smelling, tasting, and digestion.

The Cranial Bones

Eight cranial bones surround and protect the brain: the frontal, ethmoid, sphenoid, and occipital bones, and two parietal and temporal bones. They tend to be strong plate-like bones that curve to contain the brain's contours. The four bones that rise upward from the front, side, and back of the head to form the superior surface of the cranium are together called the cranial vault.

The jagged, interlocking joints between the cranial bones are called sutures. It was long thought that those joints were immobile, but functionally they are present to allow subtle movements between the cranial bones (Frymann, 1998). The individual bones move in complex spatial patterns to support the interrelated movements of the cranial sphere. If the bones do not move adequately, the sutures can fuse, but in health they move in continuous and alternating phases of flexion and extension.

The Frontal Bone: The Stargazer

The frontal bone forms the rounded anterior portion of the cranial vault, the floor for the anterior portion of the brain, and the roof of the eyes. Just deep to its anterior portion lies the frontal cortex, the part of the brain that is responsible for executive function, creativity, and the ability to respond appropriately to the environment. The frontal bone articulates with 12 bones: four cranial (sphenoid, ethmoid, and two parietals) and eight facial (two each of the nasals, the maxillae, the lacrimals, and the zygomatics). Find on yourself and on a model the following landmarks:

The frontal squama

The plates that form the forehead.

The frontal eminences or bosses

Paired symmetrical protuberances on the squama that are the original growth plates.

The brow ridges

Also called superciliary arches.

The supraorbital margins

The rim of the bone arching over the eyes.

The supraorbital notch

A small gap at the center of each orbital rim, allowing vessels and nerves to pass through.

The orbital plates

Deep to the brow ridges and above the eyes, horizontal plates forming the superior portion of the orbit. Posterior to the eye, each side forms a roughly triangular projection, to form the ethmoid notch.

The coronal suture

On the top of the head, a shallow but palpable ridge where the frontal bone articulates with the parietal bones.

Awakening the Frontal Bone

Map your frontal bone, feeling its roundness and how its frontal and upper surfaces can float upward and forward toward the sky. As your frontal bone relaxes into space, notice how the rest of your body responds. Vibrate the bone with your voice, and feel the resonance and fullness of the forward part of the skull. If you initiate movement from the awareness of your frontal bone, what kind of movement arises?

Rest the frontal bone in the palms of your hands, and let your brain rest in the cup of the bone. Relax the frontal part of your brain onto the orbital plates. Enjoy the calm and ease that provides. Breathe into the depth of the orbital plates, and even more deeply into your eyes. Let your visual perception be informed by your breath and by the relaxation of the brain and frontal bone.

The Parietal Bones: The Roofers

The symmetrical parietal bones form the sides and roof of the cranial vault. They meet each other at the sagittal suture at the top of the head, and the frontal bone at the coronal suture. They are the largest bones of the cranial vault and are basically quadrilateral. The parietal bones articulate with each other and with the occipital, frontal, temporal, and sphenoid bones. Find on yourself the following landmarks:

The parietal eminence or boss

A rounded central eminence that marks the original growth center of each bone.

The sagittal suture

The line at the articulation of the two parietal bones.

Bregma

The point at the intersection of the coronal and sagittal sutures.

The lambdoid suture

The articulation between the occiput and the parietal bones.

Lambda

The point at midline where the sagittal and lambdoid sutures intersect.

The parietomastoid suture

An irregular suture between each parietal and its neighboring temporal bone.

Asterion

The meeting point of the lambdoidal, parietomastoid, and the occipitomastoid sutures.

Embodying the Parietal Bones

Trace the surfaces of your parietal bones, and their sagittal, coronal, lambdoid, and parietomastoid sutures. Feel the four corners of each bone, to feel the dimensionality of the skull. Then with the palmar surfaces of your fingers, touch the parietal bones lightly, with the weight of a nickel. Wait patiently and breathe, feeling for the movement of the bones at the sagittal suture, widening and narrowing the distance between them. Vibrate the bones with your voice.

Breathing into your parietal bones, allow them to receive the energy of the sun and the sky. This topmost part of the head, along the sagittal suture, can be very mobile and light, to allow for the movement of the entire cranium. Imagine the parietal bones sitting on the support of the temporal bones. With those bones as a support, allow the parietals to reach up to the crown with lightness and ease.

Rotate your head, initiating by moving one parietal forward and allowing the opposite parietal to retreat back. Can the bones easily alternate the initiation? Move your head toward your shoulder, so that the parietal bone on that side begins to bear the weight of the brain. Allow the brain to fall onto the bone, and feel the rounded shape of the huge parietal bone cupping the brain. Repeat on the opposite side.

The Occiput: the Basement Organizer

The occiput is the foundation of the skull, sitting beneath the brain as part of the cranial base. Its condyles provide the support for the rest of the skull on the atlas of the spine and surround the point of entry of the spinal cord into the brain. Its motion helps to organize and balance the paired bones of the skull, the parietals and the temporals, and to organize the front and back of the skull. The occiput articulates with five cranial bones (two parietals, two temporals, and the sphenoid) and with the atlas. Find the following landmarks:

The foramen magnum

An oval opening in the occiput through which the spinal cord moves into the brain.

The occipital squama

A bony plate that rises posteriorly from the foramen magnum. With the nuchal lines, it is the only palpable portion of the occiput.

The inferior nuchal line

A horizontal ridge for muscle attachments close to the base of the occiput.

The superior nuchal line

A higher ridge for muscle attachments.

The basilar portion

The part of the occiput that extends forward from the foramen magnum, ending in an articulation with the sphenoid bone.

Occipital condyles

The articular surfaces at the base of the occiput, which transfer the weight of the skull to the vertebral column.

Embodying the Occiput

Map the back of your skull, enjoying the sensations and noticing that the back of your skull is composed of this single rounded bone, while the front of the skull is created from a multiplicity of bones: feel the unity of the back with the contrasting complexity of the front. Moving the occiput, imagine that it is another vertebral segment, carrying the continuity of the spine into the skull. Then slide the occipital condyles on the atlas, feeling its independence from your spine. Rest your occiput back into one of your hands: allow the hand to move into the bone, and then allow the bone to move into the hand.

Feel the open circle of the foramen magnum between the occipital condyles. Glide them over the concave surfaces of the atlas, releasing your tongue and the muscles of the neck. Resting your head back onto your fingertips, massage the muscles attaching to the inferior and superior nuchal lines.

The Temporal Bones: the Jugglers

The temporal bones are the agile multi-taskers of the cranium, juggling numerous functions central to our wellbeing. They protect the brain, form the center of the cranial base, and communicate between the cranial base and the cranial vault. They house the extremely delicate organs of hearing and balance; form the joints we use for eating;

and support muscle attachments for movement of the neck and the jaw.

The complexity of the temporal bone is indicated by its origin from eight separate centers of ossification during fetal development. By birth, the centers have grown together to form three plates, which merge in early life into the temporal bone. The temporal bones each articulate with five other bones: three cranial (the occipital and parietal bones of the same side and the sphenoid bone) and two facial (the mandible and the zygomatic bone). Find the following landmarks on yourself and on a model:

The squama

The flat vertical portion that forms the wall of the cranium.

The petrous portion

The large structure that forms the inferior portion of the bone and houses the inner ear. It forms a wedge between the occipital bone and the sphenoid and separates the temporal and occipital lobes of the brain. Its sharp superior ridge forms a bony strut that runs anteromedially from the area behind the ear (superior to the mastoid process) to the center of the cranial base.

The external auditory meatus

The external opening of the ear canal, which sits superior to the styloid process, anterior to the mastoid process, and posterior to the zygomatic process.

The zygomatic process

A thin anterolateral projection of bone from the squama, forming the posterior half of the zygomatic arch, just forward of the external auditory meatus. Its superior edge forms an attachment for the temporal fascia, and its inferior edge provides an attachment for fibers of the masseter muscle.

The mastoid process

A bony projection that provides attachments for several muscles of the neck. Just posterior and inferior to the external auditory meatus, it is an important reference point for palpation of the skull.

The articular eminence and the mandibular fossa

The two surfaces that the temporal bone contributes to the temporomandibular joint. Just forward of the external auditory meatus, the mandibular fossa resembles a traditional socket for a ball-and-socket joint, although functionally it is quite different. Anterior to the fossa, the articular eminence forms a gliding surface for the condyle of the mandible.

The styloid process

A thin and pointed bony projection from the base of the temporal bone. It anchors the stylohyoid ligament and a number of muscles.

Embodying the Temporal Bones

Map the surface of one temporal bone, awakening the squama, mastoid process and zygomatic processes, and auditory meatus. Give your ear a little massage and loosen the skin over the bone. Imagine the mastoid, styloid, and zygomatic processes as spokes emanating from a hub centered within the auditory meatus. Allow the wheel to rotate from this spatial support. Sense the movement between the temporal bone and all its neighbors. Repeat on the other side.

Be aware of sound falling into the depth of your temporal bones. Vibrate the temporal bones with your voice, and feel the solidity of the bone. Then block the sound by putting the tips of your fingers in the auditory meatus. Feel the vibration of the bone with your fingers, and listen to the colors of your voice coming through the bone. Releasing your fingers, can you feel the pathway for sound from the external ear through the auditory meatus and into the bone?

There is liquid within the canals of your inner ear, for both balance and hearing. Sense the fluid moving within your temporal bone when you turn your head quickly.

The Sphenoid Bone: The Great Communicator

I have a feeling that this sphenoid bone one day will teach us how to fly...I can feel the greater wings as they surge outwards and the lesser wings aloft. It is one of the hallelujahs of my skull (Bainbridge Cohen, 1977).

The sphenoid bone is shaped like a bird in flight with a central body, two sets of wings stretching across the skull, and talons reaching down toward the earth (Figure 8.8). Its many surfaces face in diverse directions, making it the most spatially complex bone of the skull. Occupying a central point between the cranium and the face, it touches each of the other bones of the cranium and many facial bones. Find the following landmarks on a model:

The body

A midline structure, its anterior surface forms part of the wall of the nasal cavity. Posteriorly, the body articulates with the occiput, and anteroinferiorly it articulates with the vomer. The superior surface forms a deep cavity, the sella turcica (Turkish saddle), to house the pituitary gland. Adjacent to the body are the optic canals, which allow the optic nerves and the ophthalmic arteries to pass between the eyes and the brain.

The lesser wings

Extending laterally from the superior portion of the body, they articulate with the orbital plate of the frontal bone, and form part of the floor for the frontal lobes of the brain.

The greater wings

Extending laterally from the inferior portion of the body, they form the middle cranial fossae with the anterior portion of the temporal bone.

The pterygoid processes

The downward-reaching talons of the bird. They are each composed of thin lateral and medial pterygoid plates that articulate anteriorly with the palatine bones and posteriorly provide attachments for the pterygoid muscles to elevate the jaw.

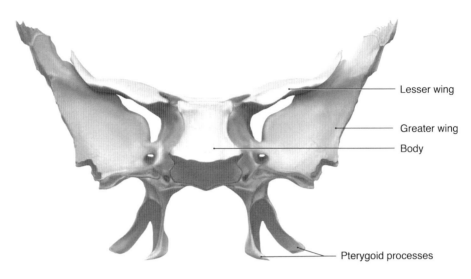

Posterior view

Figure 8.8

The sphenoid bone

Embodying the Sphenoid Bone

We can enter the sphenoid from the point of view of the pharynx in the front, from the occiput in the back, or from the greater wings at the temples. Enter your awareness of the bone from each of those directions. Can you feel the delicate expansiveness of the bone, and allow it to soar? Which bones are pushing into it? Which articulations feel compressed, and which feel free? If you release your jaw, does the balance with the temporal bone shift? If you allow the frontal bone to float, does it free the sphenoid? If you allow the parietals to rise rather than drop, how does the sphenoid react? Is the joint with the occiput free to move, or does it feel compressed? Can you feel the space behind your face, and allow the great bird to move forward into that space?

To find the body of the sphenoid, place a finger on the brow ridge of the frontal bone at midline between the eyebrows and another finger directly opposite to it on your occiput. Feel the sagittal line running parallel to the earth through your head. Then place one finger on the upper surface of each cheekbone, on little indentations just in front of your ears, sensing the horizontal that connects them. At the intersection of those two lines (sagittal and horizontal) is the sella turcica, the top of the sphenoid body, and the site of your pituitary gland. Breathe into this area and imagine the great sphenoid bird soaring.

Vibrate the sphenoid with your voice, and feel its lightness. There are two large hollows, or sinuses, within the body that provide fullness and resonance to the voice.

The Ethmoid Bone: the Hermit

The cube-shaped ethmoid is located at midline between the eyes, projecting forward from the body of the sphenoid. It has been called the beak of the sphenoid bird. Its bubble-shaped tiny cavities make it light and delicate. It articulates with more bones than any other in the skull, but it is almost entirely hidden from view, like a hermit in a cave. It articulates with two cranial bones (the frontal and sphenoid bones) and 11 facial bones (the vomer and two each of the nasals, the maxillae, the lacrimals, the palatines, and the inferior nasal conchae).

Notice the following landmarks:

The cribriform plate

A horizontal plate wedged in the ethmoid notch of the frontal bone. It forms part of the floor for the frontal lobe of the brain, and is the roof of the nasal cavity. It is perforated by many tiny holes called foramina for the olfactory nerves traveling from the nose to the brain.

The crista galli (cock's comb)

A small blade-like projection into the cranial cavity, rising along midline from the cribriform plate. It serves as an attachment for the falx cerebri, the connective tissue that separates the two halves of the brain, and separates the two olfactory bulbs.

The perpendicular plate

A flat blade at midline, forming part of the nasal septum. It articulates with the vomer and separates the two lateral ethmoid masses.

Lateral masses

Two masses flanking the perpendicular plate riddled with tiny sinuses. The lateral surface of each lateral mass forms part of the bony orbit of the eye. The medial surfaces form the upper walls of the nasal cavity.

Embodying the Ethmoid Bone

Touching the bridge of your nose, invite your awareness to flow back deep into the space between your eyes. This is the ethmoid's home and the site of your sense of smell. Feel how it flows forward from the sphenoid; the foamy spreading of the lateral masses; and how the perpendicular plate at midline reaches down into the nasal septum. Sense the crista galli rising into the cranial cavity, and its connection to the entire midline of the skull through the falx cerebri. What movement arises from that awareness?

Vibrate the bone with your voice and feel the nasal quality of the lateral masses. Keep the ethmoid vibrating, and modulate the sound by spreading the tone into other areas of the skull.

The Facial Bones

Fourteen bones contribute to the mobility of the facial structure, forming the eyes, nose, mouth, and pharynx. Facial bones tend to be smaller and more delicate than the cranial bones, and even more irregular in shape (Figure 8.9). They include the mandible, the vomer, and, two each of the maxillae, inferior nasal conchae, lacrimal, nasal, palatine, and zygomatic bones. Restrictions in their sutures and joints can result in dampened senses of vision, smell, and taste, as well as constriction in the nasal passageway and sinuses.

The Maxillae

The two maxillae form the upper face below the eyes. They provide the sockets for the teeth, the greater part of the nasal aperture, a large portion of the hard palate, and the floors of the orbits. Each maxilla articulates with two or three cranial bones (the frontal, ethmoid, and sometimes the sphenoid) and seven facial bones (the opposite maxilla, the

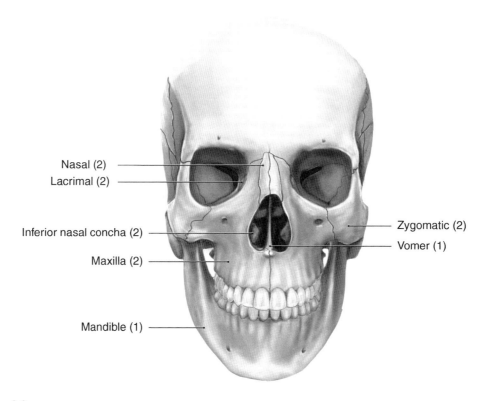

Nasal (2)
Lacrimal (2)
Inferior nasal concha (2)
Maxilla (2)
Mandible (1)
Zygomatic (2)
Vomer (1)

Figure 8.9

The facial bones

vomer, and the nasal, zygomatic, lacrimal, inferior nasal concha, and palatine bones of the same side). Four processes form each maxilla:

The alveolar process

The foundation for the roots of the upper teeth.

The zygomatic process

The foundation for the frontal aspect of the cheek

The palatine process

Forms most of the hard palate

The frontal process

Articulates with the frontal and ethmoid bones, provides a support for the lacrimal and nasal bones, and forms the orbital floor.

The Palatine Bones

The two palatine bones form the rear of the hard palate and parts of the wall and floor of the nasal cavity. They are L-shaped, the upright portion of the L forming a buffer between the maxilla and the sphenoid. Find the following landmarks on a model:

The horizontal plate

Forms the posterior third of the hard palate and the floor of the nasal cavity. Its upper surface has a ridge, the posterior nasal spine, that rises in the sagittal plane, and is smoother than the rough palatine surface.

The vertical plate

Articulates with the posteromedial wall of the maxilla and with the pterygoid processes of the sphenoid.

The palatines each articulate with six bones: two cranial (the sphenoid and ethmoid) and four facial (the maxilla, vomer, inferior nasal concha, and the other palatine).

The Vomer

The vomer divides the nasal cavity at midline, originating at the sphenoid and projecting forward. It sits above the point where the maxillae and palatines meet, forming the inferior and posterior portions of the nasal septum, which divides the nasal cavity. Find the following landmarks on a model:

Alae

Two wings that form a broad surface at the posterior end of the vomer that articulates with the sphenoid.

Perpendicular plate

A dagger-shaped projection rising from the alae, dividing the nasal cavity.

The vomer articulates with six bones: two cranial (the ethmoid and sphenoid) and four facial (both maxillae and both inferior nasal conchae).

The Inferior Nasal Conchae

The inferior nasal conchae are partially enclosed tubes that moisten and spiral the air as we breathe and participate in the sense of smell. They lie along the medial wall of the maxilla and palatines, and also articulate with the ethmoid and lacrimal bones along their superior surfaces.

The Nasal Bones

The two nasal bones are the gatekeepers of the nasal cavity. They are rectangular, standing guard at midline just in front of the more delicate ethmoid and flanked by the rising frontal processes of the maxillae. Superiorly, they articulate with the frontal bone. They are easily palpable, at the bridge of the nose.

The Lacrimal Bones

The two rectangular lacrimals are part of the medial wall of the orbital cavity, filling the gap between the ethmoid and the nasal bones, and also help to form the upper nasal cavity. They articulate with the ethmoid and frontal bones and with the maxillae and inferior nasal conchae.

The Zygomatic Bones

The zygomatic bones are the cheekbones. Each forms a spatially complex set of arches between three bones: the maxilla, frontal, and zygomatic process of the temporal bone. One rounded edge forms the lateral rim of the orbital cavity, connecting the maxilla with the frontal bone. Another V-shaped edge relates the frontal bone to the temporal bone. The most direct edge continues the forward projection of the temporal bone into the maxilla. Each of the two zygomatic bones stretches its limbs, or processes, in three directions, like an athlete reaching into space in several directions at once. Find the following landmarks on yourself and on a model:

The frontal process

The vertical portion reaching up to the frontal bone.

The temporal process

The horizontal portion reaching posteriorly toward the temporal bone.

The maxillary process

Extending toward midline it forms the lower part of the orbital margin.

The zygomatic bones each articulate with four bones: three cranial (the frontal, temporal, and sphenoid) and a single facial bone (the maxilla).

The Mandible

The mandible is the lower jaw, contributing to the action of chewing and to speech. It is the foundation for the lower teeth, provides surfaces for the muscles of mastication, and articulates only with the two temporal bones. Observe the following landmarks:

The body

The horizontal portion that anchors the lower teeth.

The ramus

A thin projection rising diagonally back from the body toward the articulation with the temporal bone.

The angle

The posterior corner, where the ramus rises from the body.

The coronoid process

A triangular projection at the anterior top edge of the ramus. It is the attachment for the temporalis muscle.

The mandibular condyle

A large, rounded articular surface on the posterior ramus that forms the temporomandibular joint with the temporal bone.

Embodying the Temporomandibular Joint

The two temporomandibular joints are unique in the body, in that they consist of two symmetrical ends of a U-shaped bone, the mandible, and two symmetrical receptacles on the skull. A moveable disc is interposed between the mandibular condyle and the temporal fossa. Movement of the disc is central to the function of the joint.

Central both to sustaining life and to communication, the temporomandibular joint is one of the most constantly used joints in the body. It supports expression by making shifts in the placement of the mandible to produce articulate speech and plays a role in the digestive system by facilitating the action of mastication. The first major accomplishment of the newborn is to coordinate sucking and swallowing, actions that require freedom and use of the temporomandibular joint.

The development of speech and language, as well as digestive tone and function, are based on that early achievement.

Temporomandibular function is central to health of the entire body for several reasons. It works in a reciprocal relationship with the atlanto-occipital joint, so restriction in either joint can cause restriction in the other, resulting in tension or dysfunction of the muscles of the neck and jaw and limitation in movement of the spine. In turn, the reciprocal movement in the temporomandibular and atlanto-occipital joints supports ease and freedom in the fluids and the meninges (connective tissue structures) of the brain.

The fifth cranial nerve, the trigeminal, innervates the muscles of the jaw. Trigeminal dysfunction will affect the jaw, and problems with the jaw will likewise affect the nerve. Dysfunction originating in the temporomandibular joint has the potential to disrupt many other systems in the body, resulting in complaints as diverse as headache, seizure activity, autoimmune disorders, digestive issues, and problems with proprioception, hearing, smell, and taste.

Finally, tension or lack of movement in the jaw can result in limitation or restriction of the soft tissues of the tongue, neck, and vocal apparatus, creating problems with vocalizing, breathing, and swallowing.

Joint Structure

Each temporomandibular joint is composed of three major elements: the condyle of the mandible, the temporal bone's mandibular fossa and articular eminence, and the articular disc between them. They are synovial joints with joint capsules, but the articular surfaces are made of tough fibrocartilage rather than the hyaline cartilage typical of synovial joints.

The Mandibular Condyles

The condyles are thick, log-like cylinders sitting perpendicularly to the mandibular rami at their ends. Wider than deep, their lateral ends, or poles, are nearly continuous with the lateral surface of the rami, but the medial poles project inward a considerable distance. The poles of the condyles do not sit on the horizontal dimension, but travel medio-posteriorly. Lines following the axis of medial-lateral poles of each condyle will intersect just anterior to the foramen magnum.

The Temporal Surfaces

The mandibular fossae of the temporal bones sit just forward of the external auditory meatus. At rest, the mandibular condyle nestles in its concavity. The fossae look like deep sockets for a ball-and-socket joint. While this is true in the first few degrees of movement, the bone at that surface is extremely thin, inappropriate for supporting a powerful joint. When the jaw opens significantly there must be a forward translation of the mandible: the condyles do not remain in the fossae but glide forward onto the articular eminence just anterior to them. The eminence is composed of stronger trabecular bone, and is actually the primary pressure bearing surface for the joint.

Feeling the Temporomandibular Joint

Place your fingers just inside the ear canals. Pressing anteriorly, open your mouth very slightly, and feel the rotation of the condyles within the fossae. As you open your jaw wider can you feel the condyles moving forward? As you close your mouth can you feel them returning to their place in the fossae?

Try opening your mouth while touching the lateral surfaces of the condyles, limiting their motion to rotation within the mandibular fossa. How does that feel? Where else in your body do you feel this motion? Then open your mouth again, this time guiding the condyles forward in space along the articular eminences. Which sensation do you prefer? Which feels easier?

The Discs

The temporomandibular joint depends upon a mobile articular disc between the two bones. The disc has two functions: it provides a concave socket on its lower surface for the rotation of the condyles, and it provides a concave gliding surface on its upper surface for riding over the articular eminence. The disc thereby maintains the continuity of function in the jaw. The concavity that forms a hinge joint with the rounded condyles of the mandible remains the socket for the condyles throughout the jaw's movement, as the disc glides forward and back along the articular eminence. The upper surface of the disc excursions around the convexity of the articular eminence.

Movement of the Temporomandibular Joint

The temporomandibular joint complex permits in movement in six directions. The movements represent different combinations of rotation in the lower joint and gliding in the upper joint. Functionally, these motions combine to create complex variations to serve sucking, chewing, swallowing, and speaking.

Mandibular Depression

Mandibular depression is the opening of the mouth. In the initial stages of opening, the condyle rotates in the lower joint, then the upper joint glides forward, and the disc slides anteriorly on the articular eminence as the distance between the lower and upper teeth increases.

Mandibular Elevation

Mandibular elevation is closing the mouth. It reverses the process of depression.

Mandibular Protrusion

Mandibular protrusion is jutting the jaw forward in space without opening the mouth. All parts of the jaw move forward at the same rate, in symmetry, and there is no condylar rotation, only gliding on the upper joint.

Mandibular Retrusion

Mandibular retrusion is sliding the jaw backward without opening the mouth. It reverses the process of protrusion.

Lateral Deviation

Lateral deviation is sliding the lower teeth to either side. This occurs when the condyle of one side spins in the lower joint while the condyle of the other side glides forward on the upper joint, resulting in the movement of the chin to one side. (When combined with asymmetric elevation and depression, this motion is central to chewing and grinding food.)

Joint Coordination

Imagine a marionette speaking by flapping its jaw, its neck and skull held still with only the mandible moving. That is distal movement of the temporomandibular joint. Imagine eating and talking that way all the time. Some people do. It tends to restrict motion, create tension in the surrounding structures of the throat and neck, and constrain the breath.

Proximal movement of the temporomandibular joint occurs when the jaw is stabilized and the mouth opens and closes in relationship to a stable jaw (Figure 8.10). With that motion the mandibular condyles can initiate motion for the proximal temporal bones. In this movement—the skull riding over the condyles—breath is restored, ease is established in the tissues, and the motion is freer and of larger scale than with the first movement.

Furthermore, proximal movement at the temporomandibular joint requires reciprocal movement at the atlanto-occipital joint, with the occipital condyles rotating within the concavities of the atlas. This easy, coordinated motion at the two joints is the foundation of the sucking and swallowing of infants. (Watch a baby nursing, and see if its head

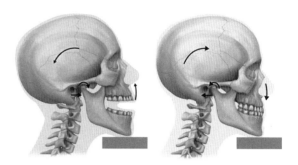

Figure 8.10

Proximal movement of the temporomandibular joint

moves easily at the atlanto-occipital joint as well as the temporomandibular joint.) We receive many benefits from maintaining or re-establishing this ease as adults.

Proximal and Distal Movement at the Temporomandibular Joint

Distal Movement

Place your fingers on your cheekbones to inhibit movement of your skull. Open and close your mouth (depressing and elevating your jaw) without allowing the other joints of the skull and neck to respond to the movement. Try speaking with this marionette-like hinged jaw. How does that feel to you?

Proximal Movement

Place your fingers on your jaw (or your jaw on a table) to stabilize it in space. Open and close your mouth, elevating and depressing the jaw, without letting the mandible move in space, forcing movement into the cranium. Feel that your cheekbones and upper teeth are rising away from and descending toward your lower teeth and jaw. (This can be very difficult for some people!) Notice how that movement requires participation at the atlanto-occipital joint. What happens to your neck, your breath, and your body as you do this? How is it different from distal movement?

Then initiate the same movement (opening and closing of the jaw) with awareness of both joints—temporomandibular joint and atlanto-occipital joint—participating. What sensations or awareness does that motion create? Now bring your intention to the supporting bone of the joint, the atlas, and initiate the rocking of the atlanto-occipital joint from there, using proximal initiation of distal movement. As you do that, relax the temporomandibular joint, allowing it to open and close as a result of the proximal initiation at the atlanto-occipital joint.

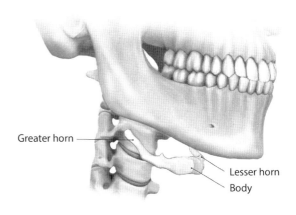

Greater horn

Lesser horn

Body

Figure 8.11

The hyoid bone

Embodying the Hyoid Bone

The delicate hyoid is the only bone in the body that is not directly attached to another bone (Figure 8.11). It is a horseshoe-shaped half-ring that floats at the junction of the neck and the jaw. Forming the skeletal base for the tongue, it is suspended by ligaments from the styloid processes of the temporal bones. Muscular and ligamentous structures radiate from the hyoid to the cranium, mandible, tongue, larynx, pharynx, sternum, and shoulder girdle. Because of its multiple and spatially complex attachments, the hyoid is part of a tensegrity structure, where deformation at one point will result in change at other points.

The hyoid is composed of five major portions. Ossification among the five portions is not complete until midlife. The five portions are the following:

The body

Sitting at midline, the body is the slightly curved center portion of the horseshoe.

The greater horns

The greater horns form the two ends of the horseshoe, reaching posteriorly and slightly laterally from the body. The tip of each horn is a rounded tubercle, the attachment for the thyrohyoid ligament. Early in life, a cartilaginous articulation joins the horns to the body.

The lesser horns

Two small cones that project superiorly from the upper surface of the bone near the point where the body and the greater horns are joined. They serve as an attachment for the stylohyoid ligaments. Prior to ossification, the lesser horns are connected to the body by fibrous joints.

Locating and Moving the Hyoid

Touching the angles of your jaw with the index finger and thumb of one hand, allow them to slide a little bit down and anteriorly from the angles. Resting your fingers on the skin, depress one side slightly and then the other. Feel for the tubercles of the greater horns of the hyoid. Be very gentle, and do not press; let your touch descend through the layers until you find a bony presence. It may help you to move your head and neck into slight extension. You may need to shift several times before finding the spot.

Once you have a sense of the hyoid's shape and location within yourself, initiate small movements from the bone. Rotate it to the right and left, letting your head follow along. How does that affect the sensation of head rotation? Let your hyoid depress a little to the front, and allow your head to follow along. Let your hyoid elevate a little from neutral, allowing your head to follow along. How do these movements affect the muscles and sensations of your neck and head?

The hyoid plays an important role in speech. It supports the tongue in its articulation, the vocal diaphragm in its vibration, and the trachea and lungs in the process of breathing. Releasing tension in muscles around the hyoid releases tension in the vocal cords and the muscles of the larynx. Bringing awareness to the alignment of the hyoid, in relationship to all of those structures, can create powerful support for the postural alignment of the head, neck, and trunk.

Postural Support from the Hyoid

Imagine a friend standing in front of you, their arms outstretched in a gentle rounded embrace. Then imagine that your hyoid is that friend, and that the greater horns are outstretched arms reaching toward your spine. Sustain the embrace of the hyoid toward your spine and notice what happens. How are the muscles of your tongue, neck, and shoulders affected? What happens to your breath and your digestive tube? What happens with your vision? How does your spine feel, particularly in the cervical area, and how does it affect the balance of curves in your spine?

The hyoid supports the passageway for breath, because the thyroid cartilage and the trachea descend directly from its inferior surface. The hyoid also protects the passageway for food leading to the esophagus, and provides attachments for muscles that contribute to the action of swallowing.

Hyoid Release with Partner

With your partner sitting or lying supine, position yourself at one side, with easy access to the neck and head. Place one of your hands to the back of your partner's upper neck. With the other hand, locate the hyoid bone with your thumb and index finger. Touch the surface of the skin over the greater horns of the hyoid, but do not press into the area. Be aware of the bone underneath, but do not force your touch into your partner, as this can be a very sensitive area. Focus on your breathing and on your partner's breathing. From that base, follow any movement or gliding that you feel through the skin.

With one hand on your partner's neck, move the other hand to the underside of the jaw. Invite your partner to breathe into the thick base of the tongue, and to feel the length and width of the underside of the jaw, flowing back into the hyoid bone.

Flying with Six Wings

Beginning a class on skeletal integration some years ago I invited the group to image that each body cavity—the head, the chest, and the pelvis—contains a pair of skeletal wings. We found that the sphenoid wings help the head orient in space, the scapular wings allow the arms to float, and the great wings of the pelvis help the body fly across the earth. One of the participants, a rabbi, returned proudly the next day with this verse from the bible, Isaiah Chapter 6, Verse 2:

Above him stood the seraphim; each one had six wings;
with two he covered his face, and with two he covered
his feet, and with two he did fly.

(A seraph is an angelic being that flies near the throne on which God is seated.) Since that time I have imagined that each of us has within us an angel with sphenoid wings to modulate our senses, pelvic wings that embrace our feet, and scapular wings for flying!

Furthermore, I realized that each set of wings relates to a center of wisdom: the head-brain for the sphenoid, the cardiac brain for the scapulae, and the enteric brain for the pelvis. I saw that each set of wings is energetically supported by a pair of endocrine glands. The pituitary, ensconced in the sella turcica of the sphenoid body, is the rider guiding the sphenoid (like Daenarys Targaryen on her dragon) with the pineal gland balancing it from the back; the thymus and the glandular aspect of the heart help the scapular wings and arms to embrace space; and the coccygeal and perineal bodies are energetic centers that help to mobilize the pelvis and legs.

Flying with Six Wings

Locate the sphenoid bone within your skull. Walking in space, allow your sphenoid wings to create lift, forward and up. Then allow the wings to elevate and depress, inviting your head and body to follow along wherever the sphenoid wants to fly.

- Enliven your special senses—vision, hearing, smell, and taste—as the sphenoid moves you, and allow the sphenoid bird to explore the environment.

- Locate, breathe into, and awaken your pituitary and pineal glands. Let them give direction and vitality to your sphenoid wings.

Then mobilize your scapulae: map them by pressing a small ball into them or have a partner touch them. Imagine your scapulae as wings and your arms, hands, and fingers as feathers, letting the movement of your scapulae guide your arms through space.

- Incorporate your heart's wisdom into the movement. Feel how your scapulae, arms, and hands support the needs and desires of your heart, moving into and out of relationship.

- Breathe into the glandular energy of your heart, letting it expand and flow through your blood toward your hands. Move the thymus beneath your manubrium, awakening its passion and allowing it to support the radiant quality of your scapulae. Tap it, vibrate it with your voice, and observe how it enlivens your wings.

Map the iliac wings of your coxal bones, through touch or the pressure of a ball. Individuate the two halves of your pelvis and feel the role of each wing as you move. Your legs, feet, and toes are feathers; let them brush the earth as your pelvic wings impel you through space.

- Let your enteric brain, the intelligence of your small intestines and colon, give purpose to the pelvic wings. The enteric brain moves us toward safety and reacts to danger—feel the satisfaction of safely completing an obstacle course.

- With your breath and voice enliven the tiny energetic structure at the tip of your tail, the coccygeal body. Invite its radiance to relax your hip joints. Add breath and vibration in your perineal body at the base of your pelvic floor between your anus and genitals (in Taoism the point is called Hui Yin, in yoga it is related to muladhara). Let the energy of the perineal body ground through your legs and feet to allow the pelvic wings to fly.

Take some time to explore the six wings and allow your imagination to fly.

Somatic Practice and Pedagogy

The beauty of a somatic movement practice is that we can apply the knowledge to our own self-development, to working as educators with individuals, and to working with groups and within communities. With creativity, somatic explorations can easily be integrated into existing dance, yoga, or exercise classes: with training, time, and experience it is possible to teach somatic movement education as a self-contained discipline outside the frame of other practices. If you are interested in somatic movement education and therapy as a profession, the International Somatic Movement Education and Therapy Association's approved training programs provide excellent training, each one with a slightly different focus and point of view (*www.ismeta.org*).

The word education can sometimes arouse the memory of negative experiences as students in hierarchical educational systems. We are too often conditioned to think that we know little, and that our inborn wisdom is of little value. The teacher is in a position of power, and owns the knowledge. Many of us retain emotional or psychological damage from our schooling, so in somatic movement we want to establish a model of learning that is empowering and respectful of the learner. The word educate has within it the root *ducere*, "to lead," and the prefix *ex*, meaning "out." According to its etymology, education has the potential to be leading, enticing, and non-invasive. As somatic movement educators, our responsibility is to guide people into relationship with themselves, and to re-awaken their innate self-knowledge and their body's internal organization. We support them in contacting themselves at the

deepest levels, and harvesting their insights so that both guide and students are engaged in exploration and learning. As educators, we provide information, maps, techniques, and support for the process, but we follow the wisdom of our students or partner's body.

The magic of engaging in this process from the embodiment of the skeletal system is that bones provide a sense of containment, clarity of form, and organization that can be applied both to guiding groups and individuals. Your personal skeletal embodiment can provide you with valuable tools for organizing yourself as an educator.

Pedagogy

Pedagogy is the science of education.

When we first start guiding others through the principles and material of somatic awareness, it is easy to think that simply presenting the material is enough. We need to remember that what we are really doing is facilitating a process of people coming home to their bodies. The material, such as presenting the anatomy and function of the tarsal bones, is only the means to that end, not the goal. For most people anatomic details and somatic principles are not important. It is the experience of self-discovery that is the heart of our work, and we need to be sensitive that our personal interests in the minutiae of anatomy or a particular image do not overwhelm our students. Use the specifics to entice your students and support your teaching of embodiment, but try not to confuse the goal of embodiment with the details. Ideally, what you are sharing is some part of the essence of your self, and what the student discovers is some essential aspect of their being.

Skeletal Principles in Teaching

Whether you are teaching dance, yoga, an academic subject, a martial art, or somatic movement education, skeletal principles that inform the movement of your body can also support your communication with students. Maintaining awareness of how support precedes movement and other principles can enhance the educational experience both for you as teacher and for your students.

Support Precedes Movement

If you want your students to achieve a specific goal or learn a new skill, anticipate the underlying knowledge and elements that need to be in place as building blocks for the skill. Students will be able to move into new territory only when the stable foundations for that movement are in place. Think backwards from your goal and carefully anticipate all the foundational elements that need to be in place for your students to attain the educational objectives.

Contents and Container

Be clear about what you are presenting (the contents), and don't lose the thread of that material. Try not to confuse the material itself with the structural container of the class. For instance, a teacher of yoga or dance may state that a class concerns breath, but if excessively challenging movement is presented that interferes with or diminishes awareness of the breath, then the content of the class, the breathing, has been lost. In that instance, it would be preferable to acknowledge that the class is about asana or movement skills, with a complementary focus on breath, but not to assert that breathing is central to the class.

The container aspect of a class may encompass many different things, including its structure, the pedagogical traditions of the discipline, the physical space of the room, music, and even the way people are arranged in space. We need to make sure that all those containing aspects of each class support the central idea, the contents.

Mobility and Stability

A stable learning environment is predictable and safe. It uses repetition as a mode of learning, places an emphasis on the teacher's role as the focus of the class, and constantly reviews older material as new material is introduced. Mobility in learning has to do with associative thinking, unpredictable or surprising teaching techniques, and keeping students off-guard in order for them to experience themselves in new ways. The emphasis is on the student experience, and the teacher follows the interest of the group.

Both styles have advantages and disadvantages. How do you balance these qualities in your classes?

Awareness of the Planes

Horizontal plane awareness in teaching uses interpersonal relationships (in small or large groups), creative projects and processes, and emphasizes the dynamics of the group as a tool for learning. Horizontal plane awareness creates a relational resonance in the mind of the room.

Vertical plane awareness in teaching emphasizes presenting, lecturing, evaluation, assessment, listening, and discussion. Vertical plane awareness creates a discursive resonance in the mind of the room.

Sagittal plane awareness in teaching encourages learning through action, movement, vocalizing, hands on, and other explorations. Sagittal plane awareness creates a goal oriented, active resonance in the mind of the room.

Planning Classes

Each teacher has his or her unique method of planning. If you already have teaching experience you certainly know already what works for you. The following are suggestions for utilizing skeletal principles to increase your range and as guidelines for those who are beginning to teach.

Embodiment

Before planning the specifics of a class, take time to make sure that you are embodied in the material you wish to present. Your teaching will partly occur through resonance—allowing the students to learn by resonating with your own personal engagement with the material. You do not have to have completely mastered the material before you teach, but it needs to be deep in your bones before you share it with others.

Shaping a Class

Skeletal awareness provides support for the architecture of a class. What form will you provide the students for their learning? Shaping can have to do with time (creating a clear beginning, middle, and end), with space (varying the directions, the configurations, the numbers of people working together), and with energy (the overall phrasing of a class, such as low tone to high tone to low tone). Successful classes can have many shapes. A common form for movement classes, which can be applied to many other types of classes, has four phases:

*   A warm-up phase, which aligns the teacher with the students and the class members with each other

*   An introductory phase of presenting basic material A deepening phase of more intense physical activity and mastery

*   A cooling or resting phase at the end.

The Outline

It is very helpful to have an outline—a skeleton—for each class you teach: it is your safety net. It is equally important to seize opportunities when they arise in class to diverge from the plan and follow the interest of the group. A class plan can be as simple as a few notes, reminding you of material you want to cover, or as complex as a written menu with the details of each exercise, exploration, or idea you intend to present.

Transitions

Transitions between activities and ideas are the joints of your class. In our bodies, we need to provide consistent and even space to the joints, allowing energy to flow from bone to bone. We need to do the same in our classes, by providing space for students to breathe and reflect within the transitions between activities. Carefully planned transitions can help to make meaning of the information you share in each activity. This might be simply inviting your students to take a time of reflection on what they have doing before you move on, or changing the tone of the room by introducing a surprise element—a prop, a visual image, or by using space in a new way.

Group Assessment

You may have created a wonderful plan for a specific class, but when you arrive you find that it does not match the students' energy level, or that you have too small or large a group, or that there is some other problem with your plan. In that case, you will have to problem-solve quickly, retrieve what you can from your plan, and proceed in a different way. Even in cases where there is not an extreme gap between the nature of your plan and the conditions of your class, assess the group you will work with at the beginning of each class to see what subtle adjustments you might need to make. Match the tone of the group, meeting them where they are in that moment, and gradually shift the tone or energy to support your original plan. Meeting their tone establishes trust: when trust is established there is willingness to flow with you toward learning.

Teaching Learning, Learning Teaching

Sharing material that you are currently learning or exploring is one of the best ways to make discoveries about yourself, the material, and your students.

Your primary responsibility as a movement educator is to facilitate your students' learning experiences. You can discover new aspects of the material with them. Don't be afraid to share your process.

Conversely, when you are sharing material that you have thoroughly embodied, make sure to utilize the class to learn something new. Your learning may be tangential to the material, but try to record your observations the way a scientist would record research. Perhaps you make a new connection, or observe students responding to stimulus in a new way, or the class will generate a question for further investigation. In this way, each class can recycle into fresh planning for the next class, and your curiosity will be aroused rather than deadened by the repetition.

Teaching Skeletal Material

When guiding somatic movement education classes (for instance a class on the bones of the foot), there are several additional considerations. The process of somatic movement education requires both cognitive and experiential learning, and achieving a satisfying balance of these learning processes can be challenging. Consider the wide range of options available to you in facilitating a skeletal class. These include:

- Movement
- Hands-on
- Guided sensory explorations (somatization)
- Lecture and discussion
- Small group activities (three to five people)
- Sounding
- Creative expression (dance, singing, painting, making music)
- Small group discussion and processing (two to three people)
- Music
- Props and play.

Notice which options you gravitate toward habitually and try to explore using options that are more of a challenge for you. Students have different learning styles and rhythms, so the more varied and dynamic you are able to make your classes, the more individuals you will be able to reach effectively.

Props and Teaching Aids

It is important to use your imagination in bringing examples, props, visual materials, and other aids into teaching. Use the things that make most sense to you personally, and which you enjoy working with. Several basics, such as a skeleton model, are essential in teaching the skeletal system, and there are many additional options. Suggested aids include the following:

- Articulated skeleton
- Disarticulated skeleton (individual bone models)
- Examples of real bone, if possible
- Anatomical images, via books or projection
- Music for movement.

Other objects that have been used by teachers include:

- Joint models
- Clay for making bone models
- Tensegrity toys
- Kneepads and braces to temporarily immobilize joints
- Architectural images
- Cogwheel toys
- Wooden snakes to show the spine.

Somatic Practice with Individuals

Working with partners in somatic movement education dyads, we listen, observe, and feel the whole person. We use the skills and knowledge we have developed in movement facilitation and hands-on techniques to address the needs of others, develop curiosity, and support transformation where it is needed. Each student or partner needs individuated responses from you, appropriate to the moment and respectful of your relationship. When you trust the process and yourself, your guidance can be very direct and powerful. Developing that trust, and remembering that the work lives within you, enhances your effectiveness as a guide.

Having embodied the skeletal material of this book, you have some skills to begin practicing with other people. Your toolkit includes each exploration you have done as well as new explorations that you will devise through your own curiosity.

A good way to begin working with other people is to follow your primary personal interests. Your repertoire will expand as you learn to address the needs of individuals who present you with unfamiliar issues. You may improvise your responses or address their needs through further study, but it is important to use each new partner's specific needs as a learning opportunity. Use the following suggestions to support yourself in transforming from the "I'm not sure what to do" mindset to being curious, confident, and responsive in your practice sessions.

Shaping a Session

Each somatic movement session with a partner has several phases. The order of events will vary, based on the dynamics of the relationship. Some of the phases will be distinct and others you may experience as constantly overlapping waves or cycles that are always present and necessary. Consider the following elements as the building blocks of an educational session you do with an individual:

- Meeting
- Observation and assessment
- Session planning
- Agreement
- Beginning the work
- Improvisation and exploration
- Communication
- Re-evaluation
- Closure
- Transition and summary.

Meeting

The moment you come into contact, your guidance begins. Your partner is the subject of the dyad, so provides the contents for the session. As the guide you are providing containment, so allow the embodiment of your bones to be a support for the moment you meet. At that moment of meeting, you are being observed and felt by your partner on many levels—some conscious and some unconscious—and your skeletal grounding, your clarity, and your organization are the foundation of the relationship.

Meeting is also your time for information gathering. Determine what form of intake best suits your style as a somatic movement educator. Do you have a checklist of questions that you ask each new partner? How do you engage them in speaking about their needs and desires for the session? What does your partner want to improve, investigate, or change about their present state?

Observation

Observation is ongoing within a session, but at the outset needs to encompass the question "Where is my partner in the present moment?" Your observation can be made through tracking movement habits, by listening to expressed needs and goals, and by attending to the feeling tone of your partner's expression rather than to the specific content. Your observation within the session also includes information you receive while touching: what is the underlying tone and how does it change as you provide awareness in the tissue?

Session Planning

This phase needs to answer the questions: What can I offer this person? What is the best use of our time together? Where can we start? What material do we want to cover? What are my goals in supporting ease and transformation for this person? These questions should be discussed and a clear intention for the partnership should be articulated. This establishes the spine of the session. You may also consider questions of stability and mobility: do I support the person where they are in the moment or do I support change?

Agreement

The agreement phase is often made in the process of session planning, but you should think of it as a distinct and separate phase. Have you made clear agreements to establish the container for the session? For time? For movement? For touch? For the degree of intimacy or privacy required? For support in emotional processing? Clear agreements on those issues help to create trust and safety.

Beginning the Work

Following session planning and making agreements, it is helpful for both parties to be clear about the moment in which the session begins. If the session is to begin with movement, help your partner to enter their own physicality after the verbal exchange. If the session is to begin with touch, ensure that your partner is comfortable and that you are centered and clear in yourself. Only then begin your exploration together.

Improvisation and Exploration

After your exploration has begun, you may continue as planned or the exploration may yield unexpected results that will tempt you to diverge from your plan. (The most important material often lies beneath the surface and cannot be anticipated.) Begin with your plan but allow the relationship to develop organically. Your partner's responses in the moment may well change your approach and the plan. Dancers and musicians develop the skills to improvise from a score or an outline. Your session plan is your score and you are free to utilize the tools of improvisation to alter and change it. The improvisation phase is where you may become aware of different rhythms and phrasing within a session. It is always possible to diverge from the spine of the session to follow a limb, a logical outgrowth, and eventually return to the spine of the session.

Most works of art have a form, whether it is a piece of music, dance, theater, or an object from the visual arts. You can think of your session as a work of art, and see what form emerges. As your interest and curiosity yield new information, be mindful to continually refer to your original agreement and ensure that you are not violating it as your work of art takes on a life of its own. Embracing your own skeletal embodiment will help you to sustain a sense of clarity and purpose during the exploration.

Communication

Communication can be a distinct phase of the session or an ongoing dialogue, but it is essential for you as the guide to take responsibility for maintaining communication about what you are doing. Lack of communication can result in assumptions being made on the part of the guide, and the partner feeling lost. When someone goes deeply inward and loses the desire to communicate, a skilled guide can offer open-ended questions or observations that do not force the partner into unwanted communication, but will still yield valuable information for the guide.

Re-evaluation

Re-evaluation can also be either an ongoing process or a pause in the session to assess whether the original agreement is still in force, whether the session plan needs to be changed, and whether a new assessment needs to be made.

Closure

The guide needs to take responsibility for bringing the movement or hands-on session to a clear ending. Questions, emotions, or ideas may linger or be incomplete, but the time frame of the session demands that you help your partner to feel a sense of completion in the moment, even when there are incomplete aspects. This can take the form of large movement, full-body touch, discussion, or other integrating techniques.

Transition and Summary

Be sure to leave enough time in the session to allow your partner to transition to pedestrian life. This transition process should include time for them to express what the experience has been during the session. It is part of the learning process for both the partner and the guide.

Forming Sessions with Skeletal Themes

As you integrate information from other body systems and developmental movement into your knowledge base, your options for addressing movement from a skeletal perspective will expand and your ability to utilize skeletal touch and principles to support other concerns will increase.

This book has offered various tools, principles, and techniques for skeletal embodiment. By consciously collecting these tools and applying them to your work with individuals, you will find that your repertoire in somatic movement education is already quite expansive. Table 10.1 offers examples of how you can apply the explorations to your work with others and how you can organize those explorations into educational themes that might address the needs of students.

Three Magic Words

As you embody your skeleton and help others to do so, you are engaging in the culturally subversive act of experiential learning—listening deeply to the wisdom of your own body in relationship to the world, rather than to information that is imposed on you from the outside. You will relax into the trust that your experience of the environment is first in the tissues, the bones, the body, and then taken up and interpreted by, rather than controlled by, the conscious mind. It is the foundation of somatic movement education.

As you develop your practice of experiential learning with others, you can take inspiration from those three magic words: somatic, movement, and education. Somatic awareness, as defined by Thomas Hanna, is the study of self from the perspective of lived experience, encompassing the dimensions of body, psyche, and spirit. Movement is the most important sign of life, encompassing both the pattern of vibration that holds matter together and larger movements of the human body: at every level its essence is transformation. Education is leading someone toward the light of awareness. Simply put, we use mindful movement—the process of embodiment—to guide others toward transformation in all the layers of their being. It is the most satisfying work I know, and embodying the bones is a wonderful point of entry.

Table 10.1: Themes, Issues, and Explorations

Theme	Issues Addressed	Possible Explorations
Establishing weight flow through the spine	Addresses various types of back, neck and hip pain, alignment problems, and breath constriction. Supports ease of relationship with the earth.	1. Standing Forward Roll Downs (Chapter 8, page 146) 2. Establishing the Spinal Curves (Chapter 8, page 147) 3. Weight Flow Through the Discs (Chapter 8, page 154) 4. Seated Weight Flow Through the Spine (Chapter 8, page 155) 5. Spinal Tap (Chapter 8, page 156)
Mobile foot and stable foot awareness	Addresses pronated or supinated feet; ankle, knee, and hip problems; and gait. Supports balance of mobility and stability.	1. Mapping the Rays of the Foot (Chapter 4, page 46) 2. Mobile Foot and Stable Foot: Standing and Walking (Chapter 4, page 49) 3. Mobile Foot/Stable Foot Standing Alignment (Chapter 4, page 50) 4. Dividing Mobile Foot and Stable Foot (Chapter 4, page 50) 5. Walking the Railroad Tracks (Chapter 5, page 85) 6. Standing Toes to Pelvic Half (Chapter 5, page 89)
Atlanto-occipital and temporomandibular joint coordination	Addresses neck and jaw tension, back pain, organ dysfunction, hypertension. Supports general health.	1. Establishing the Spinal Curves: Locomotion (Chapter 8, page 147) 2. Finding Yes and No (Chapter 8, page 150) 3. Atlanto-Occipital Mobilization (Chapter 8, page 150) 4. Embodying the Occiput (Chapter 8, page 160) 5. Feeling the Temporomandibular Joint (Chapter 8, page 167) 6. Proximal and Distal Movement at the Temporomandibular Joint (Chapter 8, page 168)

Table 10.1: (Continued)

Theme	Issues Addressed	Possible Explorations
Relationship of shoulder girdle to dome of ribs	Addresses neck and upper body tension; nerve and blood flow to upper extremities; shoulder, elbow, and wrist restrictions; supports reach into space.	1. Mapping the Shoulder Girdle (Chapter 6, page 116) 2. Shining the Dome (Chapter 6, page 129) 3. Compression and Release: Ribs and Sternum (Chapter 6, page 129) 4. Resting the Shoulder Girdle (Chapter 6, page 117) 5. Shoulder Girdle Mobilization (Chapter 6, page 118)
Skeletal relationships between fingers and scapula	Addresses integration of upper limb and torso, balances movement in the shoulder joint and shoulder girdle, brings space to joints of arm and hand.	1. Mapping the Shoulder Girdle (Chapter 6, page 116) 2. Mapping the Hand (Chapter 6, page 96) 3. Pleasure and Ease (Chapter 7, page 135) 4. Embodying Lines of Connection: Fingers to Shoulder Girdle (Chapter 7, page 138)

References

Bainbridge, Cohen B.B., Leeds R., Kalab L., Peffley, S., Wylie K., 1977. Skeletal System: Manual for a Workshop in Body-Mind Centering® (unpublished manual). Amherst, MA: The School for Body-Mind Centering®.

Bainbridge Cohen, B., 1995. Self-Study Guide to the Skeletal System (unpublished manual). Amherst, MA: The School for Body-Mind Centering®.

Bainbridge Cohen, B., 2018. Basic Neurocellular Patterns: Exploring Developmental Movement. El Sobrante, CA: Burchfield Rose.

Berland, E., 2017. Sitting: the physical art of meditation. Boulder, CO: Somatic Performer Press, pp. 49–54.

Bradley, K., 2009. Rudolf Laban. New York, NY: Routledge, pp. 106–112.

Dimon, T., 2011. The Body in Motion: Its Evolution and Design. Berkeley, CA: North Atlantic Books

Douglas, E. and Fitzmaurice, C., 2004. Interview with Catherine Fitzmaurice. Available at: https://static1.squarespace.com/static/5569e19fe4b02fd687f77b0f/t/5a754963085229a6161ecdb6/1517636311816/Douglas-Fitzmaurice+ActingNow+Interview+2018.pdf, p.3 [Accessed 10 October 2018].

Eddy, M., 2016. Mindful Movement, The Evolution of the Somatic Arts and Conscious Action. Bristol, UK: Intellect.

Franklin, E., 2003. Pelvic Power: mind/body exercises for strength, flexibility, posture, and balance for men and women. Hightstown, NJ: Princeton Book Company, pp. 18–22.

Frymann, V., 1998. The Collected Papers of Viola M. Frymann, DO. Ann Arbor, MI: Edward Brothers, Inc., pp. 17–30

Greenleaf, D., 2017. Reflections on the skeletal system [letter by email] (Personal communication, 24 April 2017).

Hartley, L., 1995. Wisdom of the Body Moving: An Introduction to Body-Mind Centering. Berkeley, CA: North Atlantic Books.

Juhan, D., 2003. Job's Body: A Handbook for Bodywork. 3rd ed. Barrytown, NY: Barrytown/ Station Hill Press.

Levangie, P. and Norkin, C., 2011. Joint Structure and Function: A Comprehensive Analysis, 5th ed. Philadelphia, PA: F. A. Davis Company, pp. 229–232.

Massa, N., 1559. Liber introductorius anatomiae [online]. Venice. Available at: https://web. stanford.edu/class/history13/earlysciencelab/ body/skeletonpages/skeleton.html [Accessed 27 March 2018].

Mitchell, H.H., Hamilton T.S., Steggerda F.R., Bean H.W., 1945. The Chemical Composition of the Adult Human Body and its Bearing on the Biochemistry of Growth. Journal of Biological Chemistry, pp.158–625.

Nandikeshvara, 2nd century AD. Abhinaya Darpana [online]. Available online at: http:// onlinebharatanatyam. com/2007/11/28/abhinayain-dance/ [Accessed: 27 March 2018].

Bibliography

Bainbridge Cohen, B., 2012. Sensing, Feeling, and Action, 3rd ed. Northampton, MA: Contact Editions.

Bassam, C., 2018. Fitzmaurice Voicework®. [online] Available at: http://cynthiabassham.com/fitz_Interview.html [Accessed 26 March 2018].

Biel, A., 2014. Trail Guide to the Body, 5th ed. Boulder, Colorado: Books of Discovery.

Bradley, K., 2008. Rudolf Laban. New York, NY: Routledge.

Franklin, E., 2003. Pelvic Power for Men and Women. Highstown, NJ: Princeton.

Frymann, V. M., 1998. The Collected Papers of Viola M. Frymann, DO: Legacy of Osteopathy to Children. Indianapolis, IN: American Academy of Osteopathy.

Hackney, P., 2002. Making Connections: Total Body Integration Through Bartenieff Fundamentals. New York, NY: Routledge.

Hartley, L., 1995. Wisdom of the Body Moving, An Introduction to Body-Mind Centering. Berkeley, CA: North Atlantic Books.

Hoppenfeld, S., 1976. Physical Examination of the Spine and Extremities. East Norwalk, CT: Prentice-Hall.

Houglum, P., Bertoti, D. and Brunnstrom, S., 2012. Brunnstrom's Clinical Kinesiology. Philadelphia: F.A. Davis.

Ingber, D., 1998. The Architecture of Life. Scientific American, 278(1), pp. 48–57.

Johnson, D., 1995. Bone, Breath, & Gesture. Berkeley, CA.: North Atlantic Books.

Juhan, D., 2003. Job's Body: A Handbook for Bodywork. 3rd ed. Barrytown, NY: Barrytown/Station Hill Press.

Kahle, W., Leonhardt, H. and Platzer, W., 1992. Color Atlas and Textbook of Human Anatomy. Stuttgart: G. Thieme Verlag.

Lesondak, D., 2017. Fascia: What it is and Why it Matters. Edinburgh, UK: Handspring Publishing.

Levangie, P. and Norkin, C., 2011. Joint Structure and Function: A Comprehensive Analysis. 5th ed. Philadelphia, PA: F. A. Davis Company.

McHose, C. and Frank, K., 2006. How Life Moves: Explorations in Meaning and Body Awareness. Berkeley, CA: North Atlantic Books.

Milne, H., 1998. The Heart of Listening. Berkeley, CA: North Atlantic Books.

Netter, F., 2014. Atlas of Human Anatomy. 6th ed. Philadelphia, PA: Elsevier.

Olsen, A., and McHose, C., 2004. Bodystories: A Guide to Experiential Anatomy. Lebanon, NH: University Press of New England.

Palastanga, N., Field, D., and Soames, R., 2013. Anatomy and Human Movement: Structure and Function. 6th ed. Burlington, VA: Elsevier Science.

Pischinger, A., 2007. The Extracellular Matrix and Ground Regulation: Basis for a Holistic Biological Medicine. Berkeley, CA: North Atlantic Books.

Schuenke, M., Ross, L., Lamperti, E., Schulte, E. and Schumacher, U., 2006. Atlas of Anatomy. Stuttgart, New York: Thieme.

Tortora, G. and Grabowski, S., 2000. Principles of Anatomy and Physiology. New York: John Wiley & Sons.

Tsiaras, A. and Werth, B., 2004. The Architecture and Design of Man and Woman. New York: Doubleday.

Weintraub, W., 1999. Tendon and Ligament Healing: A New Approach Through Manual Therapy, Berkeley: North Atlantic Books.

White, T., Black, M. and Folkens, P., 2012. Human Osteology. Amsterdam: Elsevier Academic Press.

Index